BIOHACK YOUR WAY BEYOND LYME

BIOHACK YOUR WAY BEYOND LYME

AN INSPIRED GUIDE FOR RECOVERY

LISA RUDY WILLIAMS

FREEWORKS
PRESS

DISCLAIMER
No part of this publication may be reproduced or transmitted in any form or by any means, mechanical or electronic, including photocopying or recording, or by any information storage retrieval system, or transmitted by email without permission in writing from the author.

Neither the author nor the publisher assumes any responsibility for errors, omissions, or contrary interpretations of the subject matter herein. Any perceived slight of any individual or organization is purely unintentional.

Byproduct names are trademarks or registered trademarks of their respective owners.

The author of this book does not dispense medical advice or prescribe the use of any technique as a form of treatment for physical, emotional, or medical problems without the advice of a physician, either directly or indirectly. The intent of the author is only to offer information of a general nature to help you in your quest for health and well-being. In the event you use any of the information in this book for yourself, the author assumes no responsibility for your actions.

Published by Freeworks Press
Lisa Rudy Williams Wellness Management, LLC
1930 Village Center Circle, Suite 3-139
Las Vegas, Nevada 89134

ISBN 978-1-949165-22-7

Editorial work and production management by Eschler Editing
Cover design by Steven Novak
Interior print design and layout by Marny K. Parkin
eBook design and layout by Marny K. Parkin

This book is dedicated to:

MY GRANDFATHER, PAUL,

who cheered me on, supported my stopping at nothing to get well,
inspired me to overcome great obstacles, and motivated me to keep
getting better every day in every way. I am so grateful for you.

MY HUSBAND, GEOFF,

who stood by me through thick and thin, carried me at times,
provided either tender care or tough love when I needed it most,
and grew with me on this journey. I love you for everything.

MY GUARDIANS, ABBY AND LEIA,

who both saved my life, got me out of bed and made me walk,
protected me from harm, and restored my faith in the Universe.
I would not be here without you, and I feel eternally blessed.

CONTENTS

FOREWORD

H ealth is the most valuable resource we have at our disposal. For those with Lyme disease, co-infections, and other autoimmune conditions, however, achieving optimal health is their greatest challenge. This is now compounded by the current world crisis and the unprecedented unease it brings. Thankfully, individuals still have the power to take back control when they understand the true causes of illness and use appropriate biological treatment methods to restore good and vibrant health.

Having practiced medicine in the United States since 1982, I have long been aware of the limits of conventional medicine in properly diagnosing and treating Lyme disease. There is little understanding of how chronic toxicity affects the health of the body and contributes to pain, autoimmune diseases, and autonomic dysfunction. Rather than address the root causes of disease manifestation, conventional approaches focus on treating symptoms. The biological medicine I learned in Germany and the Eastern medicine I learned in India taught me that an integrative approach to treating disease is necessary for the body to heal.

Over my more than forty years of practice, I have seen many different types of patients walk through my door. Since I mostly see the sickest of the sick, they are all desperately in need of help. However, not all patients who come to see me are as determined to survive and recover as Lisa was. She overcame tremendous obstacles on her journey back from late-stage Lyme disease and I, along with her other doctors, have encouraged her to write this book for several years. It is a gift to see her doing so well, and I know she will help the many people who read this book.

Biohack Your Way Beyond Lyme is unlike any other book for people trying to recover their health. What is unique about Lisa's message is that she focuses on how important one's mindset is when it comes to healing and how it empowers people to seek answers and solutions outside the conventional model of medicine. She creates a vision of what is possible and motivates patients to pursue a new approach that will move them beyond their current reality. This book is very timely for those who are seeking novel methods for recovering from illness and taking care of their personal well-being in today's toxic world. Biohacking is an approach that is relevant for any patient who is dissatisfied with mainstream medicine. More than ever, we can all benefit from adopting a biohacker's mindset in confronting the many health challenges we face at this time in history.

This book addresses some of the important concepts in biological medicine I have been teaching physicians and patients throughout my career: the importance of addressing the root causes of disease, testing the body for autonomic dysregulation, and taking action to eliminate the toxins and hidden infections that contribute to chronic illness. However, Lisa does not stop there. Throughout the book, she discusses the idea that it takes more than the medical interventions themselves for Lyme patients to fully recover. She discovered that getting well required transforming her beliefs about herself and adopting a different identity to move beyond her long history of illness.

Biohack Your Way Beyond Lyme is written for the patient who is struggling with their health and ready to embrace new ideas. The book is written to help people at a time when their symptoms feel overwhelming and they need a message of hope and inspiration. Lisa explains some very basic scientific information in easy-to-understand ways and in a conversational style, making the book very accessible and a quick read. She really does know what her audience needs because she has been there.

I hope you are motivated to pursue a greater level of health after reading this book and inspired to take a stand for your liberty during a time when governments are making decisions that affect your freedom as an individual. Keep those biohacking principles in mind as you step into the empowered role Lisa envisions for you. When you embrace that vision for the future, you are well on your way to recovery.

—Dr. Dietrich Klinghardt, MD,
Founder of the Sophia Health Institute, Woodinville, WA,
Head of the Klinghardt Institute
Online International Training Program, UK, 2020

INTRODUCTION

"In a time of drastic change, it is the learners who will inherit the future."

—Eric Hoffer

What does it mean to biohack? Essentially, the word *biohack* means to experiment on your own body. A biohacker is someone who seeks to improve their health by upgrading their personal biology. The brave new world of biohacking is an exciting frontier for those who want to explore the full capacity of the human body. You can think of it as do-it-yourself biology.

The very fact that you were attracted to this book tells me you are a visionary person. I celebrate and honor you for being curious. That is the true quality of a biohacker in the making. Biohacking is all about having a vision of infinite possibilities. It's knowing you have greatness inside. To biohack means to say yes to life in spite of everything in your present experience.

You know that Lyme disease wreaks havoc on your biology. Your body has been through a lot, but it has an innate intelligence and can heal under proper conditions. The amazing field of biohacking utilizes strategies that enhance the healing potential already at work within you.

If you have curiosity and the intention to move beyond Lyme, this book is for you. The goal of biohacking is to be able to thrive and maximize your well-being on an ongoing basis. As you biohack your way to recovery, you will learn that absolutely anything is possible for you. When you're ready for a life beyond the condition of illness, you're ready to be a biohacker.

1

"WHY ISN'T THIS WORKING?"

"When you have exhausted all possibilities, remember this—you haven't."

—Thomas Edison

Let me start by asking this: How's your life going right now? Let me guess . . . you feel like screaming, *"Nothing is going right! My life is a total shitshow! Lyme disease sucks. I can't stand it anymore."*

Does that resonate with you? I imagine it does. Go ahead and scream it at the top of your lungs if that feels good. Get it out of your system. Really, I don't mind waiting. Throw in a few air punches or beat a pillow if that helps. I hear you loud clear. It's completely understandable.

Your life, quite frankly, is really freaking hard. You've dealt with just about every symptom imaginable. You cycle through them on a daily, weekly, and sometimes hourly basis: brain fog, migrating pain, memory loss, depression, heart palpitations, headaches, seizures, cravings, upset stomach, bowel problems, stiff joints, muscle pain, vertigo, hearing and vision problems, confusion, tremors, insomnia, night sweats, migraines, and word block.

Even just reading that paragraph was a complete struggle and took all your concentration. You feel stuck in despair with your current treatment protocol as you trudge along day in and day out while your body seems to be betraying you. You can barely get out of bed sometimes. You're depleted and hurting. You can't work. Your whole identity revolves around illness.

You have nothing to give anyone anymore. You feel like you can't take care of your family or be there for your partner. You feel like you're disappointing everyone in your life. Nobody can depend on you because you cannot predict what the next hour holds.

Your brain isn't working, and your memory outright sucks. You know you won't be able to remember anything, so you try to write everything down, which is annoying but the only way you can function. It feels like you're just spinning your wheels, following along diligently with what you're told to do but never really seeing your condition change for the better.

You've been on quite a winding road to get to this point. It took a really long time to even get a diagnosis of Lyme disease, and when you did, you were just grateful to finally get an answer to the health problems plaguing you for years. The diagnosis was almost a relief because you hoped you would receive treatment and feel better in no time at all.

But that wasn't how things turned out to be, was it? You got started on some of the treatments your doctor prescribed, and you quickly learned that treating the illness meant going through times of feeling even worse than ever. You soon found out it wasn't going to be an easy journey, but you were willing to follow along with the treatment protocol, trusting that, eventually, you would feel better.

Well, it's been months or years, and you're still not feeling like your health is improving. You struggle to get through each day, just to take care of yourself. Your brain still isn't working, and your body feels like your enemy. You have the sense that you're not moving anywhere. You look at the situation and think to yourself, "What's the point? Where is this even getting me?"

You follow the treatment protocols you've been given but don't see results. You don't think they're working. You're afraid there's no hope for you. You feel like you just can't go on doing the same treatments anymore, but you don't know where else to turn.

You want a future to look forward to; it seems so bleak right now. You have no sense that things are ever going to get better. You're not even sure it's possible for you. You've been told that this is a chronic disease and perhaps it isn't even possible to recover or live a more full life.

What if I were to paint a different picture for you? A vision of the future that holds space for progress, for you to confidently say, "I'm getting better. Today is better because I'm seeing results. I'm actually doing something that's working. I see some good happening."

That's what I envision for you. That's what I know to be completely possible. Your destiny is bigger, deeper, broader, and more wonderful than a life of slow decline. A life of sickness, despair, fatigue, and neurological impairment is like being on a runaway train going downhill. It doesn't have to be that way. You absolutely can see your treatments making a real difference so you no longer feel like you're at the whim of the illness.

You *can* recover.

What does recovery look like for you? What might be possible? What if you did have the energy to do the things you want to do? What if you got up every morning with a sense of purpose, knowing you could put your life's energy into your work or your relationships with family and friends? What if you felt like your body was a resource rather than a detriment to your health? What if you had a greater sense of optimism, peace of mind, and self-assuredness?

That might seem far-fetched, but I want you to try to envision your life as if you were recovered from Lyme disease and living out your dreams. Instead of spending your time trying to plan around your treatment, imagine planning a wonderful vacation with eager anticipation or working on a project you are totally passionate about.

Rather than spending your time focused on the pain you feel in your body right now, imagine you are focusing on how good it feels as you laugh and soak up warm rays of sunshine, or dance to music, or enthusiastically pursue an ambition you have always wanted to pursue.

That future reality is my vision for you—you living a life beyond Lyme, a life in which you are functioning as the very best version of yourself. I see you healthy, strong, vibrant, connected, peaceful, joyful, and free.

You are spending your time moving toward your goals and collaborating with people you love and respect. I see you being at home in your body, trusting it to uphold you as you openly explore the world of possibilities available to you in this lifetime.

I envision you feeling confident again, knowing you have overcome the greatest conceivable challenges. You're standing tall, proud, and ready to take on new endeavors with a stronger sense of self than ever before.

Your whole body vibrates with gratitude, appreciating what you've been through to heal it. You have a voice now; it serves you well to speak your truth. This is the future I see for you. I believe with all my heart that it's not just possible; it's your destiny for this to be your reality.

I know you're afraid to even go there, to try to see yourself or your future like this. You've been disappointed before, and you'd rather not put your heart on the line again. You're really afraid that you'll never recover. It's too hard to imagine a different reality than the one you've been living.

You fear your life is just one long, downward spiral from here, that there's no hope because you'll always be sick. Your lack of success with everything you've done thus far has proven that you're stuck in this frustrating cycle. You don't want to cling to false hope or trust anybody who tells you otherwise.

I completely empathize. I'm not asking for your trust here, only your willingness to see this book through to the end. My job is to hold space for your healing as we progress through the book together. Your job is to see it through by showing up and keeping an open mind.

Can you do that? Are you willing to try? If so, then all you have to do is decide to read through this book from start to finish. In it, I will show you how to consciously move toward a life beyond Lyme and accelerate your progress in achieving a more abundant state of health.

2

"HOW WOULD SHE KNOW?"

"In order to love who you are, you cannot hate the experiences that shaped you."

—Andréa Dykstra

You probably want to know a little bit more about me before you commit to reading this book. After all, you've never heard of me, and you've listened to so many sources of information. It's hard to believe anyone can actually recover from this awful illness—it sounds too good to be true. Your particular struggles feel insurmountable, bigger than I can possibly understand. Nobody in your life gets what you are going through. So how can I?

It's true that nobody in your life gets what it's like to have Lyme. Honestly, they just can't. It's not their fault. They might love you and wish the best for you, but they can't identify with what it feels like in your body or how it's affecting you physically, mentally, and emotionally. Thankfully, I can—or I would not be writing this book. I say "thankfully" not because I would wish my experiences upon anyone but because it connects me to you on the deepest level.

By telling you a little of my history, I'm putting my faith in you. I trust you to open your heart and not just your mind, because I'm showing up for you as a real person. Like you, I have been through hell on earth. My hope is that being willing to reveal the innermost aspects of my journey will prove to you that I am willing to show up with courage on your behalf.

Over and over, I'm going to tell you that courage is the key to success, so who would I be if I didn't show up here with courage? My being vulnerable about my story will hopefully give you a picture of why I have some insight that might be of value to your recovery.

My road to recovery started with the diagnosis of Lyme and co-infections in 2012 but, like yourself, my health problems extended a long ways back. I also went through many years of being undiagnosed due to a lack of awareness of Lyme disease. When I was growing up in California during the 1980s and '90s, there was simply no knowledge of the prevalence of Lyme.

I spent much of my childhood in the outdoors of the western United States. I camped and hiked with my family, frequently getting bitten by mosquitoes and the occasional spider. Wearing shorts and sandals, I played in the orchard behind my house and ran through grassy fields where deer gathered. I thought nothing of it other than being annoyed that I was always a magnet for bug bites. This was normal to me, and being in nature was where I felt most free.

When I was bitten by a tick on the back of my head one family vacation, my parents removed the engorged parasite from my hairline, and life went on. They had no reason to worry at the time because they didn't know all the risks associated with vector-borne illnesses.

Not long after that incident, however, my health started spiraling downward. I had always been a relatively happy child, but soon after that vacation, I began exhibiting anxiety and depression, including debilitating panic attacks and obsessive-compulsive thinking.

Next, I started having symptoms that affected many different bodily systems. My hyperactive immune response resulted in severe environmental and food allergies, asthma attacks, and digestive problems I had never experienced before.

I suddenly started getting recurring sinus infections for which I was given repeated courses of antibiotics. I also developed acne and psoriasis, which I would later understand were signs of fungal overgrowth and dysbiosis in the gut. Despite seeing many different types of doctors for these problems, I was never informed as to how my diet affected my health.

As my immune system became more impaired, I ended up getting sick with a significant viral infection that caused profound fatigue. Although I was hospitalized,

I was never actually treated for the infection. I was told by the doctors that I would eventually just get over it.

During that time, I was also having gynecological problems, with excessive bleeding during menstruation and excruciating pain. Instead of evaluating the cause, my doctor put me on birth-control pills to diminish the symptoms, even though I wasn't sexually active.

Blood tests showed Hashimoto's thyroiditis, but no one ever asked what was triggering the autoimmune reaction. The specialists I saw weren't communicating with each other, and I didn't have a family physician who could link all of these systemic issues together.

The answer every doctor offered was to prescribe a pill for a symptom. They would deal with the presenting problem without putting it into a larger context. This continued for years. And I got worse without any real insight into what was going on underneath the surface.

Ultimately, my psychological symptoms became the most concerning to my parents, who didn't know where else to turn medically. After seeing several psychologists, I was referred to a psychiatrist who diagnosed me with bipolar disorder, which she called manic depression.

As a result, I spent fifteen years believing I was mentally ill and needed psychiatric drug therapy instead of infectious-disease treatment. The drugs sedated me but didn't treat the underlying problem: a brain inflamed by infection. It was the inflammation in my brain causing the anxiety, depression, and chronic insomnia.

Meanwhile, my obsessive-compulsive thinking was getting out of control. I developed an eating disorder that started with a period of anorexia and progressed to binging and purging. No matter how much talk therapy I underwent, I felt as if I was being driven to consume sugar and carbohydrates by a force within me that didn't feel like it was actually me.

Each time I gave in to these cravings, I hated myself for it and felt a strong sense of guilt and shame. But I didn't know how to stop; it was as if I had been overtaken by a physiological drive I couldn't control. I didn't even realize how impaired my digestion was because of the bulimia. I had bowel movements consisting of only undigested vegetable matter instead of stool.

Despite my young age, my body felt like it was breaking down. I had joint hypermobility, especially in the spinal column, with excessive laxity of all my ligaments. Even as a teenager, I needed chiropractic adjustments multiple times per week because my alignment wouldn't hold.

Neurologically, I was not well. I couldn't concentrate and had terrible insomnia. For many years, I took sleeping pills every night, which led to more disordered eating patterns. The sedatives and antipsychotic medications often made me sleep for more than twenty hours at a time.

What was most scary was the memory loss. I couldn't recall even basic details in my life. Often I'd forget why I was doing an activity when I was in the middle of it. I couldn't remember the names of people, places, or events from the recent past. I had virtually no long-term memory, and I had trouble finding everyday words for conversation. By this point, I had been on lithium and the other psychiatric drugs so long I thought maybe they were causing the memory loss.

Being misdiagnosed as bipolar cost me a decade that I could have dedicated to seeking real answers. But at the time, I didn't understand how infectious agents could infiltrate the brain and cause the symptoms of "mental" illness. Not getting tested for Lyme and co-infections left me in a much more advanced stage of disease by the time I was finally properly diagnosed.

Eventually, I developed heart-related symptoms that were repeatedly dismissed by emergency room doctors at various hospitals. They told me in patronizing voices that I was creating psychosomatic symptoms and that the palpitations weren't real. But I knew I didn't have a psychological problem. I had an irregular heartbeat and excruciating breastbone pain.

Rather than do more in-depth testing, they treated me like a hypochondriac who was only imagining these physical sensations. It wasn't until years later that I learned these symptoms were due to a Bartonella infection. In addition to endocarditis and inflammation of cartilage near the ribs, I had bulging veins all over my body and sometimes experienced uncontrollable rage.

I was living on the East Coast of the United States by that time and constantly getting bitten by mosquitoes, sometimes by the dozens per day. Although I was irritated by these itchy, inflamed bites, I had no idea I was being exposed to serious vector-borne illnesses, such as Bartonella, that could affect my heart, blood vessels, brain, and other organ systems.

Ultimately, it was not until my exposure to residential mold that I reached a catastrophic breaking point with my health. I didn't know about the mold contamination because it was growing inside the walls of the building I was living in, due to an undetected water leak.

Within a relatively short time, I developed constant pain in my back and legs. Soon it became so unbearable I could barely walk and had to take a medical leave from my job as a biology teacher. Despite undergoing spinal injections, acupuncture, and being on hydrocodone and muscle relaxers, I experienced no relief until I finally moved out of that toxic building.

Unfortunately, that didn't happen before my husband and I lost a baby during the early stages of pregnancy. It was devastating, and though it didn't lead directly to any answers, it led me to a doctor who eventually ordered testing for Lyme. She was an OB/GYN, and while she didn't know my extensive health history, she was open-minded and agreed it was a good idea.

By pursuing this testing, I was finally diagnosed with Lyme disease twenty-two years after the tick bite. Eventually, other test results revealed I had severe heavy metal toxicity and many co-infections. These included multiple species of Bartonella, several viruses, microscopic parasitic infections, pathogenic gut bacteria, *Candida*, and other fungal infections.

At first I thought all these discoveries would help me find me a clear path to getting well, but I quickly learned that there was nothing straightforward about treatment for these conditions. I found out that the existing medical system was in complete disagreement about how to—or even whether doctors should—treat Lyme and address the problems with the immune system.

When I disclosed I had Lyme disease on my medical paperwork, conventional doctors questioned me with unsympathetic skepticism. Even in the most renowned teaching hospitals, I was told Lyme and other parasitic infections were rare in the United States. It turned out Lyme was a controversial topic and doctors treating the illness faced scrutiny. Although I hoped I would have a clear prescription for recovery, I soon learned that wasn't going to be the case.

When I finally started treatment with an out-of-state Lyme doctor, my body was a mess. I had paralysis of the digestive tract and pain throughout my back, ribs, shoulders, jaw, hips, and neck. My blood pressure was so low I often felt dizzy. My face drooped on one side because of an infection of my trigeminal nerve, and I felt tingling throughout my mouth and sinuses.

At my sickest, I had an extreme sensitivity to environmental noise, an auditory processing disorder, and was agitated by the electromagnetic frequencies of computers, wireless signals, and cell phones. I experienced a buzzing feeling in my head that became worse at night. Sleep was nearly impossible, so I spent hours lying awake, listening to guided meditations.

My neck was constantly cracking, especially in the upper cervical region where the vertebrae surround the spinal cord at the base of the brainstem. I had severe tendonitis in my wrists, so I had to wear braces to limit their use. My muscles were always rock-hard with tension, and I only got temporary relief from massage. The spasming of my trapezius muscles kept me from raising my arms over my head and made it difficult to lift things.

When I began taking the multiple antibiotics prescribed by my first Lyme doctor, my levels of pain and anxiety skyrocketed as I was hit by the full impact of the Jarisch–Herxheimer reaction. A Herxheimer reaction, or "herx," is the body's response to the toxins released as harmful microorganisms die off during antimicrobial treatment. My body wasn't able to eliminate the toxins fast enough. I felt like I was dying. I had no idea what I was doing wrong.

I had followed the doctor's orders, assuming that I'd start feeling better, not worse. Since I'd been on oral antibiotics countless times for ear and sinus infections, I didn't expect this would be any different. I thought I would start to improve after a short time on the pills. But as I quickly discovered, being on antimicrobial treatment for Lyme disease was nothing like that.

Instead of feeling better after the first few days, I felt infinitely worse, the severity of my symptoms increasing tenfold. I even started having new problems, with rashes erupting on my skin, sweating and chills, nausea, tremors, muscle twitching, headaches, uncontrollable crying, delusional thinking, and insomnia alternating with horrible nightmares.

I was scared of what was happening and had no idea where to turn. My close family didn't know what to do, so I felt infinitely alone. I assumed the Lyme-literate doctor would have told me everything I needed to know, but he'd said nothing about this. I was on my own until I could schedule a phone consultation or hear back from him by email.

Through that experience, I learned the hard way that doctors who prescribe treatment aren't necessarily the best equipped to help their patients get through it. They may not be readily available and can't always provide ongoing support. I found out I would need to learn for myself.

I started doing research as thoroughly as I could manage with a brain that felt like it was on fire. On the internet, I found suggestions from other patients about what self-care techniques might be helpful. I decided to try anything and everything. I had no idea what I was doing, but I was desperate. It was up to me to find what was most effective.

I discovered what I needed most was to reduce the toxic load from the die-off of the infections. The more techniques I used to help my body with elimination, detoxification, and lymphatic stimulation, the better I felt, physically and mentally.

That was my first arena for biohacking: supporting my body with self-care practices and using innovative technologies so I could better tolerate treatment. I learned many strategies for reducing the toxicity, which decreased pain, increased my energy, improved sleep, and calmed my anxiety.

I found that with more elimination and detoxification support, I could stay at a higher level of treatment. This was an essential realization because it helped me see that it was *my* actions that defined my success. Although I wanted a doctor to just wave a magic wand over my body, I came to realize that I was primarily responsible for taking care of my body's needs.

Ultimately, whether or not the doctor gave me the most effective protocol in the world wouldn't matter if I couldn't stay on it. The doctor couldn't do for me what I wasn't doing for myself. As much as I wanted to be rescued from my discomfort, I was the only one who could rescue myself. I had to step into a proactive role, acting on my own behalf.

Having the ability to help my body felt good. I realized I'd never really nurtured it in this way. I gained confidence from figuring out what to do when nobody was there to advise me and started to trust my instincts for the first time in my life, rather than only look to doctors.

It became clear that if I was going to recover from Lyme, I had to be part of the solution. So I set my mind on learning everything I could to improve my health, whether it was endorsed by "experts" or not. I began to read and listen for information about treatments outside of what I was already doing. I started using other methods to achieve health and got good results.

The more I tried, the greater the sense of accomplishment I felt when I observed that my own experimentation was really useful. I was uncovering what doctors couldn't see with lab tests. I was making discoveries my doctors couldn't make with conventional treatment strategies.

Soon, my personal research led me to alternative solutions that yielded more effective results than many of the other things I had tried. When I followed my instincts, I made progress. This energized me and gave me a sense of hope about my future even though the present circumstances were painful and difficult to withstand.

Becoming a biohacker motivated me to take action. I focused on doing whatever I could and trusted that *something* would work. I called it the "kitchen-sink approach" because I was throwing all my energy, resources, and heart into my efforts and trying everything.

As I became more attuned to my body and experimented with unconventional treatments and do-it-yourself interventions, I felt empowered. I was seeing results, and I was excited to know I was co-creating my healing. This new way of thinking was what launched me into the exciting world of biohacking and transformed my vision of the future.

What I am going to offer you in this book is how my experience becoming a biohacker benefitted my health and helped me recover from Lyme. I have been on the ground, biohacking my way for many years now, doing things the conventional medical system won't even acknowledge as effective. It hasn't been easy, but it has been worth it to get to where I am now.

Biohacking has taught me that there is a limitless field of possibility when it comes to restoring your health. Even after more than twenty years of being undiagnosed, I was able to recover from Lyme, and using what I have learned, I continue to improve my health on a daily basis. If there was hope for me, there is hope for you. My desire is to help you find your path forward so that you can feel good about your progress and start living out your destiny.

3

"WHAT CAN I EXPECT?"

"And suddenly you know: It's time to start something new and trust the magic of beginnings."

—Meister Eckhart

Now that you know a little about me, let's figure out where we're heading with this book because I know you desperately want a way to get better. You're looking for direction; you don't have a clue where to go. This book is going to get you to the next phase of your healing, but it's not going to be via the route you thought you were going to take.

If I could tell you that what I did to get well is exactly what your body needs, I would give you that formula. I promise I would. I'd tell you to just follow my instructions and that would be enough for you to get well. The problem is, that's the same type of approach you've been taking.

You've been following prescribed protocols. You've been doing what your doctor says. But you still don't feel like you're making headway or getting to the level of health you desire. So we're not going to take the same approach here. If a protocol was the only thing that was going to make the difference for you, you could find that information from many other sources.

Instead, we're going to look at Lyme treatment from a different angle. We're going to look at how your entire mindset affects the outcome. I know that's probably going to drive you crazy because the last thing you want to talk about is your mindset. You've been battling this for so long you're exhausted and you don't want to think about your thinking.

But you know what? Your mindset is the very thing that can bring you energy. It's what boosts morale. It's what can change the whole trajectory of your recovery. It's the one thing that affects every decision you make about your treatment and how your body will respond.

In this book, we're going to cover how your mindset can help you have confidence in the decisions you make and take on the challenges you face with courage. This journey can be difficult, but it's how you approach the challenges that matters. It's how you think about the conditions you're dealing with and what meaning you create for yourself in the process.

You are ultimately the factor that makes or breaks your recovery—not the doctors, not the protocols. As a biohacker, you're going to be the one to decide how you approach your healing. I'm going to teach you to trust what works for your body and to use that knowledge to your advantage, knowing that you have the means to positively influence your health and your life.

What do you believe is necessary to recover? The person who gets through this illness and to the other side is someone who digs deep and trusts their inner voice. They find out how strong they are and decide that this condition is not going to define them. They intentionally create the meaning they want for their life and begin to see themselves as someone who's already healthy and whole. That's what this journey is all about and why mindset is so important.

You are powerful—more powerful than you have ever known yourself to be. As a biohacker, you're going to open up to new ideas and innovative solutions; you're going to be able to project into the future that there's a life for you beyond illness. You will see infinite possibilities, and you will stop at nothing to feel well because that is your birthright.

You are a powerful being. You absolutely have the ability to shift your health to a more positive state. Your body is designed for well-being; it is designed for having energy and feeling radiant joy. It's designed for all the good you still have waiting for you in this lifetime.

Biohacking teaches us that we can optimize the function of our bodies through life-affirming actions. It's all about the idea that our bodies truly *can* recover and be well. We each deserve abundant health, and we can indeed change the current reality of our physical existence. As a biohacker, you can take on the challenge of Lyme disease knowing you will be able to succeed when you have your full mindset behind your treatment.

The infections are something that has to be addressed. You will use your body as a testing ground to find out what works for you individually. It will take commitment to cleanse and detox your body, to hydrate and nourish it, and to support your elimination and circulation. You will need to do whatever it takes to stick with treatments that are working. Your being willing to follow through is what will make a positive difference.

In this book, I'm going to teach you how the biohacking mindset can help you recover from Lyme and set a different course for thinking about your health going forward. I have used the acronym BIOHACKER to describe the principles involved in this new way of thinking. I'd like you to read through the steps in order, from B to R. Once you have the framework, you'll be using each of these principles simultaneously.

As you adopt the mindset of a biohacker, you will start becoming the person who successfully overcomes illness. You will soon see yourself on the other side of these experiences, looking back, standing tall, observing what you have accomplished, and feeling proud of the person you've become because and in spite of them. This is the vision I am holding for you.

This is not going to be your typical Lyme book. This is not just another protocol book. This is a guide for navigating your individual treatment journey and moving beyond Lyme. It will help you gain confidence and motivate you to dig deeper than you may have gone before.

I ask only that you read all the way to the end to see where it leads you. No matter what protocol you're on, this book has a place for you because your success is all about the attitude you bring to this journey. You can do this! You *can* recover from Lyme disease, and becoming a biohacker is the way to do it. So let's get started.

4

B: BUCK THE SYSTEM

"Remember that you not only have the right to be an individual, you have an obligation to be one."

—Eleanor Roosevelt

To change our approach to treating Lyme, we have to know where we're starting from. Have you ever heard the definition of *insanity*? It's doing the same thing over and over again while expecting a different result. So let's start there. Let's first look at what isn't working for you, what's not getting you the results you want. From there, we'll figure out where to go.

The approach you've been using involves thinking that doctors know it all and that you know nothing; they know what's happening in your body better than you do. Is that necessarily true? Or is that just what you've been told all of your life? Maybe that's what you were always led to believe—that the doctor knows best. You can't possibly be the expert in your own health. How has that paradigm worked for you so far?

When it comes to Lyme, doctors have differing opinions about what works and they prescribe treatments accordingly. However, their ideas may be limited by their own biases and/or medical training. Perhaps they rely on peer-reviewed research in medical journals as a guide for treating their patients. The protocols they use are designed for the "average" patient.

Well, are you the average patient? Do the published scientific studies describe your exact situation? Probably not. My bet is that your situation is pretty unique. I'd predict that most doctors haven't been able to answer what you feel needs to be addressed.

So let's stop the insanity and start thinking differently. It's time to stop putting your faith in everybody else and start putting some of that faith in yourself. It's time to start thinking of these medical personnel as consultants supporting you.

The doctors, nurses, therapists, and other trained specialists are going to be helpers alongside you, but you're going to become the lead decision-maker. You're going to start taking back the power of your self-knowledge. You're going to trust your inner authority.

This is going to be the framework for what I call "bucking the system." Bucking the system doesn't mean you stop everything you're doing now. It doesn't necessarily mean you fire all your doctors, although it may mean that. It means you start taking responsibility for every decision that gets made. You want your power and your voice to be the lead voice.

The first time I made a choice to buck the system, it was both scary and empowering. After ten years of psychiatric drug treatment, I woke up and realized it wasn't working for me. It wasn't addressing the underlying causes of all of my health problems. What I needed was for somebody to look deeper. What I needed was for somebody to be an investigator.

I respectfully fired my psychiatrist and decided to start my own hunt for answers. Instead of continuing to go along with a program I didn't believe in at my core, I said, "You know what? I don't know what the answer is. But I know this isn't the answer. This isn't the answer for me, so I'll be on my way. Thank you very much. Bless you. I will move forward on my own."

Even though I didn't feel prepared to move forward on my own at the time, I knew I needed to start charting my own course. I had to find doctors who would investigate with me, not ones who told me that because they didn't know the answer, there was no answer to be found.

That was bullshit, and I knew it. That was just their egos getting in the way. They couldn't admit that they didn't know. They didn't have a beginner's mind, and that's what I really wanted. I learned that I needed to get rid of the people who were not the right fit for me.

When you buck the system, you don't stop doing what's working for you right now. Instead, you take inventory. You look at the doctors and people you're already working with and ask, "What is their intention for me? Do they think they already know all the answers? Or are they open to new ideas and solutions? Do they invite my curiosity?"

As you reflect on your experiences with these people, stop and ask yourself, "Do they try to find answers to my questions? Do they discuss treatment options in a collaborative way? Do they listen to my concerns in the way I deserve to be listened to? Do they reflect back what they've heard me say? Do they acknowledge me as the decision-maker?"

When you form a team of medical personnel and health consultants, your job is to guide them as to how you want to be treated. You start by standing up and telling them what you need. You can do so with kindness and set a clear agenda: You want to make your own decisions. You want to be informed. You get to make the calls for your own body. *It is your birthright to do so.*

Once I stepped out of mainstream medicine, I found doctors who respected my judgment and valued my curiosity. They got excited when I brought them possible solutions. These are the types of people you want on your team: people you feel really good about working with.

It is so important to your treatment success that you establish a voice for yourself. You are the ultimate authority when it comes to you. You have the right to speak up. Not doing so is a surefire way to become a submissive patient. A submissive patient is a people-pleaser who doesn't want to rock the boat.

That is not who you're called to be in this precious life of yours. What you're called to do is to rise up in your power and take ownership of your health by thinking for yourself. Having a submissive attitude actually suppresses your immune system.

The medical system is filled with doctors who proclaim their authority, but, often, they don't know what they're talking about or lack integrity. Instead, they are motivated by kickbacks from profit-driven industries like Big Pharma and Big Food / Agriculture. Mainstream medicine is focused on symptom treatment because that's where the profit is. There is no profit to be made from curing people of their health problems.

That system is broken. It is a way to keep people coming back. The more symptom-treatment that is prescribed, the more side effects people have from the pharmaceutical drugs. It's the ultimate hamster wheel. We can't rely on that medical system anymore for true health care.

It's no longer the case that only certain people, like doctors and trained scientists, know all the answers. We are now living in the age of information. We have the internet and updated knowledge at our fingertips continuously. We can search online for anything we want. We can research for ourselves. Knowledge is no longer reserved for the Ivory Tower.

The traditional medical system is based largely on egotism rather than on enlightened awareness. Many doctors are stuck in an egoic state; they've done so much medical training they truly believe they know it all. It's true they've done a lot of training and may have years of experience. It's also true they bear a tremendous burden taking care of patients every day and that their jobs are highly stressful. But operating from a place of ego blocks a person from being willing to admit that he or she doesn't necessarily know all the answers.

It is your responsibility as a biohacker and consumer of health information to seek the truth and align yourself with practitioners seeking truth themselves. You have to evaluate whether the advice you receive is offered with a fullness of heart or from an ego.

You probably feel that internally when you're working with a doctor. You can sense whether the person is coming from a heart-centered or ego-centered place. The ego-centered doctor gives you a bad feeling because you feel patronized. You want a partner, not a patriarch.

Biohacking is all about stepping into a new role with respect to health care. Yes, doctors go through years and years of training. I believe most doctors are fundamentally good and have the intention of helping their patients. But that doesn't mean they know everything. Doctors are only human. Just like everybody else in life, they do the best they can at the time.

It's also true that many in the medical establishment have conflicts of interest. They don't have your highest good as their intention. They are not to be trusted with your health decisions. As a biohacker, you have the freedom to choose for yourself. You have authority over your body. Nobody else is going to stand up for your well-being the way you can and must do.

Bucking the system means first letting go of what's not working for you. It may mean leaving behind doctors who don't have the kind of energy you're looking for. You're the team leader now. You're the one who's going to make the call when it comes to your health decisions.

What you want is to draw together a team that can collaborate with you in a supportive way. This may include working with your primary care doctor, or it may require you to find a Lyme-literate doctor outside your geographic area. You might decide to consult with someone who is trained in naturopathic, osteopathic, homeopathic, integrative, or functional medicine.

Your team may include chiropractors, acupuncturists, physical therapists, colon hydrotherapists, and massage or lymphatic therapists. It may include a health coach or possibly a dietician if you can find one who is open-minded. You may find you need a team that includes other kinds of practitioners as well, both for physical and emotional support.

When it comes to working with doctors, it is your sovereign duty to speak up and ask for what you need. But you also don't want to be annoying. I say this with the utmost love and affection. Not only have I been that annoying patient, I have observed plenty of other annoying patients in doctors' offices and treatment clinics.

In these relationships, it's all about the energy you bring to the table. I like to think of annoying patients as parasites, which is ironic because a lot of them *have* parasites. But it seems that the most annoying patients are the ones who act like parasites. They're the "blood-sucking" type who drains the life out of their doctors. They're so needy, insistent, and pessimistic they actually create a really negative dynamic with the doctor.

You want to be heard without being somebody doctors don't want to work with. The key is to be an assertive patient without sucking the life out of your doctor or their personnel. The best way to do this is to keep an attitude of gratitude for the help you receive and to express that gratitude as often as possible.

You can also give them encouragement; their job is so hard. They're dealing with very sick people and are doing their best to help them. When you can be a light in their world, that's when they want to sign your lab slips. That's when they want to write your prescriptions. That's when they volunteer to help you find resources. That's when they are willing to be your partners.

In addition to working with doctors, you want to establish a support network you can regularly access for troubleshooting. As you start navigating your own treatment journey, you may find it helpful to have a community of like-minded biohackers. That way it's not incumbent on you to know everything, especially not with your current state of brain fog.

Surely you don't want to have to learn everything on your own. What an unnecessary burden that would be! We all like having people to brainstorm with and bounce ideas off. Working together in a team environment inspires and elevates everyone involved. Collaboration carries with it a powerful energy.

Remember that, ultimately, the first step to becoming a biohacker must be to buck the system. You have to let go of what doesn't serve you anymore and replace it with what feels right. When you stop relying on outside "experts" as the voice of authority, you start designing your own system of healing. You get away from the traditional approach of mainstream medicine. That's when you stop treating symptoms and actually start addressing underlying problems.

In this new role, you no longer tolerate being patronized because you deserve to be heard. You are the submissive patient no longer. You respectfully stand up for yourself. You know you are fully capable. You are now the lead decision-maker co-creating with a team of partners who supports you. Becoming a biohacker is about stepping into the light of a new age. You are free to seek truth. You have the right to make your own choices. You are bucking the system.

5

I: INVESTIGATE FOR YOURSELF

"Faith and doubt are both needed—not as antagonists, but working side by side—to take us around the unknown curve."

—Lillian Smith

Once you begin to step into your power by bucking the system, it's time for the next principle of biohacking. Don't worry, you're ready. You're the lead decision-maker now, and you know who you want on your team. You've seen how the medical system doesn't always serve your best interests, and you're imagining how you'll work within and around it to get your needs met.

Congratulations! You're already starting to think like a biohacker. So, what next? How do you proceed with designing a treatment plan that's right for you? Well, the next step is to start investigating. In this chapter, we're going to talk about expanding your ideas on what the possibilities are: what treatments, therapies, interventions, strategies, and "hacks" are out there.

We're also going to talk about how to think critically about the information you get. How can you know what's reliable and what isn't? What's truth and what's propaganda? Your job as a biohacker is to become more informed so you can evaluate the information for yourself.

I get it. It sounds overwhelming. Your brain isn't firing on all cylinders as it is. You feel like you can't interpret the things you learn about. You've looked at books and blogs and social media; you've listened to online summits and podcasts. It all goes in one ear out the other.

Let me take this opportunity to reassure you; the only thing you need for this step is already inside you. I know this because you've made it to this chapter. You clearly have the desire to recover, and you're motivated to look at a new approach. You have curiosity.

Being a biohacker requires only that you want to learn. You don't need to have a great memory. Learning happens with repetition. Do you remember being a student? Did you know everything the first time you read it or heard it? No. You repeated it and repeated it.

With biohacking, you're going to be involved in a process of ongoing inquiry. It will mean some legwork. It will mean being willing to listen to new information and reading what you can. Don't worry, reading will get easier! I couldn't read more than a few sentences at a time for more than ten years. I promise that as you recover, the ability to read comes back.

Being a biohacker does not require you to be educated in any traditional sense. You don't need to be trained in science; you will learn how to think like a scientist as you go along. All you need is the motivation to learn. And what better motivation is there than your vision for the future?

You know that what you've been doing hasn't worked for you, so now it's time to start looking at what other possibilities are out there. It's time to start opening your mind up. There is limitless potential for healing. What treatments are you interested in? What else is out there? Perhaps there are solutions you've never heard of. How will you know if you don't investigate?

The more ideas you entertain, the more likely you are to discover solutions. Investigating for yourself means you're going to start becoming aware of your preconceived ideas. We all have beliefs we've been fed from outside sources: from other people, from the medical establishment, from marketing ads, from the things we read and the conversations we hear. As a biohacker, your job is to start questioning everything and looking deeper.

The first thing you want to ask as you investigate is "What is actually truth, and what is propaganda?" So much in the news and online is not reliable. It's promoted to push an agenda or product. You simply cannot accept the things you see on television or social media at face value. It's especially hard when you're feeling desperate not to get swept up by marketing.

How do you avoid falling into that trap? First, you have to affirm that no one has the right to hypnotize you without your consent. You must decide you won't get caught up in emotion or false hope; don't let anything put you in a trance and take away your power. Stay vigilant.

But what about when the information seems to come from a credible source? For example, say it's a person with lots of degrees. It's tempting to think someone with a laundry list of credentials is trustworthy, but they can have an agenda that's not in your best interest.

When you have brain fog, it's easy to think these people are more intelligent than you are, but that's just another trance. Having more degrees can actually limit a person's thinking if they never question how they were educated. You'll have a deeper level of intelligence if you question things.

As a biohacker, you want to become a skeptic. What is represented as "fact" may not be accurate. You have to be skeptical in this age of media bias and hidden agendas. Skeptics are people who don't trust everything they see. What they do is keep a beginner's mind. They want to learn for themselves rather than have blind faith in what they hear.

It's natural to be skeptical about propaganda; you get a bad feeling when you sense dishonesty. But what about scientific research? It's important to know that even researchers are biased. Every human being has preconceived ideas and assumptions they're not even aware of. Since doctors and scientists are human beings too, their biases affect their work.

The information promoted by mass media doesn't necessarily tell the whole story. It's driven by profit. Mainstream medicine is funded by the pharmaceutical industry; dietary advice is funded by the big food companies. So you have to look at motives and conflicts of interest.

When you encounter information about health claims, ask yourself the following: How is this claim supported? How current is the viewpoint? What does the person or company have at stake? Where is the funding coming from? What is the relationship with industry or government?

Don't let yourself get overwhelmed here. Take a deep breath. The only thing you have to do is take off any rose-colored glasses that aren't serving you. You are breaking out of the trance of mainstream medicine and mass media. You're seeing for yourself now.

To get well, I did a lot of investigating. I listened to podcasts and online summits. I read online posts, blogs, and journal articles. Even though reading was hard, I bought tons of books. At first I had no idea what they were talking about. But I learned some of the terminology as I went along. I thought of it as graduate school and tried to keep a beginner's mind about everything.

That's how I want you to start. Everything is a possibility when it comes to biohacking. Because you don't know what options are going to work for you, just keep an open mind. You are a unique individual. This means what works for you might not be what's right for other people and what works for other people might not work for you.

There may be conventional treatments necessary for your recovery. Many options can really improve the health of a patient with Lyme disease. Over the years, I frequently utilized antibiotic and antiparasitic treatments. I believed they were going to help me, and they did. Thank goodness for the medications that saved my life and helped me get well.

But I also researched and used a tremendous number of alternative therapies. I did many things that weren't even on my doctors' radars. Those alternative therapies often sounded like they held just as much promise as traditional medicine, but with fewer or no side effects. I investigated every treatment, even things that were totally out of the mainstream, as an equal opportunity for improving my health.

Being a biohacker is all about getting out of the box and letting go of your limited thinking. Biohacking opens the doors to a whole new world of health and human potential. By being inquisitive, you learn not to take anything at face value. Instead, you ask questions and do the research yourself.

You start to learn how other people are doing things. You get excited about new ideas. Being an investigator means that sometimes you're going to come up with solutions nobody else agrees with because they haven't tried them. Maybe it even sounds crazy to them.

Science is all about being curious. Being a scientist means you launch out on your own sometimes, despite opposition. Other people may think your ideas sound bizarre or that those ideas couldn't possibly work. Are you going to trust them, or are you going to trust yourself?

Your family or friends might try to tell you that untested treatments aren't reliable. They might try to dissuade you from researching for yourself because they are still putting all their faith in mainstream medicine. They believe in always following the "standard of care" because that's all that they know. But are you going to listen to them or do what's right for you?

Ultimately, you're the lead decision-maker. You have to be ready for the fact that not everybody is going to agree with you. Other people may not want their ingrained belief systems to be overturned, which is totally fine. That's their business. Your health is your business. You don't have to sacrifice your rights to life, liberty, or privacy. You are an autonomous being.

When you face questioning from your loved ones about your treatment and health choices, it can be helpful to explain what you're doing and why, if they have a genuine curiosity. However, some people will challenge you with a barrage of questions solely to discredit your choices.

This was a matter I had to navigate carefully. I was truly open to any intervention that might help me recover, but there were people who questioned my decisions— everything from my treatment approach, to my diet, to my choice of doctors was controversial.

It's inevitable that you will face judgment, criticism, or doubt when you decide to step out of the conventional model. So how do you handle resistance from people when they push back against your approach? You must set boundaries around how and what you communicate. You can't allow yourself to get sidelined by detractors or waste energy trying to explain yourself.

Biohacking sometimes means going against the grain. As a biohacker, you are free to investigate whatever you want. Your path to healing is individual. You are totally unique. You've already tried what hasn't worked. It's time to start thinking outside the box.

There may be options you haven't tried. What else can you imagine is out there? If you choose to look at all possibilities with equal curiosity, you are ready for the next step: seeing your journey as that of an explorer venturing into the unknown.

6

O: OWN YOUR JOURNEY

"Don't be satisfied with stories, how things have gone with others. Unfold your own myth."

—Rumi

Okay, we've gotten through bucking the system and becoming your own investigator. Now it's time to start identifying what this journey means to you. This concept is probably the most important part of what's going to carry you through the next several steps. The meaning you bring to this journey is what defines how empowered you feel. The vision you have of yourself is what matters here. It's time to start seeing yourself as the person who recovers.

What has your thinking about your journey been like so far? My guess is that you have felt very disempowered.

You have felt helpless, even hopeless, at times. You've gotten defeated, not wanting to continue on. Lyme feels so unfair.

You know what? You're right. It is unfair. You have been suffering a tremendous burden. You deserve a better existence—one much greater than you have been imagining. But the current reality is that you are in this situation; it sucks. You are not to blame for the condition you're in right now. What you are responsible for is what you do about it.

You see, it's not about what happens to us, it's about how we respond. It's about what we do in the face of what we are dealt. That is what defines us and who we become. What can we do in the face of this illness? How do we respond? How can we define what our journey through Lyme means in a more positive way?

For a long time, my thinking was doing nothing for me. At least it wasn't helping me in any way. It was making me suffer, actually. The story I was telling myself went something like this: I am a victim of a tick bite. The doctors have all failed me. Nobody understands what I am going through. My father doesn't care. People have abandoned me. I'm missing out on everything in life. My body is broken. My gut doesn't work. My joints won't hold. I'm housebound—practically tethered to a bathroom—because of treatment. I "can't" eat, drink, or do what other people do.

I was telling myself a pretty terrible story all the time, and I didn't even realize it. Those low-vibration thoughts made me feel depressed and disheartened. No wonder my body felt awful. I was believing the worst about my situation. And I believed what other people were saying about my future: Lyme was "chronic." This projection was a life sentence that felt like a death sentence.

Does this sound familiar? We all go through this phase of thinking in the beginning. We feel like our diagnosis is a personal tragedy. How can everyone else around us have such "easy" lives? What did we do to deserve this? We get stuck in a cycle of constantly thinking about our symptoms, our pain, and our problems. We keep reiterating the story of our past and focusing on our limitations in the present. We exist in a victim consciousness that becomes our identity.

Why is this so important? When we have a victim mindset, it's debilitating to our bodies. We react to these thoughts without even knowing it. They are happening subconsciously all the time, and our body is "listening." The way we think and talk about Lyme programs our body in either a positive or negative way. Believing you're a victim of this illness is a surefire way to stay a victim and to make your body believe it's not going to be able to come back from it.

When anyone gets a diagnosis of Lyme or any disease, they construct an entire reality about it in their minds. They listen to other people's predictions and form expectations about the outcome. This happens as they go through treatment as well. They hear experiences from the other patients, read posts on social media, and listen to the opinions of every doctor, specialist, therapist, and "expert" out there. It all affects what they think.

So how can you figure out what's going on with your thinking? You start by observing what kinds of emotions you're experiencing on a daily basis. If your emotions are negative, you know your subconscious thinking isn't positive. Your thoughts are generating those negative emotions.

Observing your thoughts from a distance through mindful awareness can be useful. Some people do this in seated meditation, but I could never sit comfortably when I was really ill, so I did a lot of walking meditation in nature. Being outdoors helped me to get outside my head.

Mindfulness simply means being aware. You watch your thoughts as they happen. You don't "do" anything except notice them; you don't try to change them during that time. The whole point is just to see what shows up. By observing them with curiosity, you can be detached.

If that doesn't work for you, it may help to write things down or listen to yourself speaking aloud. What you tell someone else about your "life story" reveals how you think. You can uncover a lot through journaling, but it may work best to talk to someone who has a sympathetic ear. We all need to feel seen and heard. It's usually best to talk to someone other than a family member or friend who is an important part of your life. You'll tend to be more open and honest.

What's the story you're telling that person about your life? Who are you in the context of what you're going through? How do you frame your story: from the past, present, or future?

The idea of storytelling is important in our lives. If you look at social media, it's people telling their stories. Their stories have importance, which is why they spend so much time crafting photos and creating a narrative about what's significant to them. They're creating a story about who they are and what meaning their life has.

To recover from Lyme, you're going to need to start mentally creating the story you want to be true. You can start by asking, "What has my thinking done for me so far?" Has it motivated you? Inspired you? Made you think of yourself as strong and creative? Given you inner power? Or has it made you feel depressed, demotivated, even defeated?

You can choose to think of yourself however you want. You can choose to think of yourself as a victim of your condition—or you can believe something else. The victim story tells your life one way. But *you* craft that narrative.

You can choose to suffer or not, depending on how you think about your circumstances. For example, a person can be in physical pain without thinking of it as suffering. We can see ourselves as transcending the pain. We can see ourselves as being tough enough to sit with the present moment, see ourselves being strong through it. When we do so, we're not a victim of it.

How do you see yourself right now? Who are you, really? Who are you at the very core? What are you apart from this illness? I'd like you to find something positive about who you are beyond Lyme disease. What is one strength you have? What is one gift you have? What is one special thing you bring to this planet?

Got something? Tell me about it. Is it a skill? A character trait? That's what makes you, you. That's what makes you unique. That's what makes you amazing. Guess what? We need more of that. We need you to share your uniqueness with the rest of us. We need you here to bring more of that to this world because only you can bring it.

What else are you beyond Lyme disease, underneath Lyme disease? That's what we need more of. If you stay sick, you will never manifest more of that, but if you are determined to recover, you can bring more of that to this world. When you set a definite intention to get well, that's what you're going to bring us. You have a purpose here. We need you to be well.

Part of becoming a biohacker is seeing yourself as your own hero. You're going to start thinking of yourself differently. Lyme disease—with all its affiliated conditions—is your challenge. You were given this challenge not to weaken but to strengthen your character.

Visualization can be very helpful here. You may wish to cut out inspirational pictures, create an online vision board, or just spend time imagining yourself as the superhero in your own movie. You get to be the producer and lead actor. You get to cast yourself as the hero rising to meet the challenge. You get to see yourself moving beyond a life of limitation and disease.

What makes a hero rise up? A hero rises up when they look within and know the challenge is a test that's necessary to reach the destination. When a hero encounters trials on the journey, that hero develops the capacity to bear them and move forward in spite of them. That hero survives incredible difficulties and keeps going. That hero becomes the person who makes it through.

You're heading out into the unknown, into the wilderness, to discover your truth. That's how you can see yourself as a biohacker. You're exploring new frontiers. You're a pioneer. You're trying things out for yourself and looking at variables no one else has looked at before.

The biohacker sees it as an adventure, exciting and scary at the same time. Both can be true because, really, aren't anxiety and excitement two sides of the same coin? Aren't the things that are most scary also slightly exciting? For example, when you are standing at the edge of a steep cliff or taking a spontaneous road trip to a new place, those can be both thrilling and daunting. Anytime you do something unfamiliar for the first time, it's always a combination of emotions.

When I first started biohacking my health, I was nervous and excited about everything I learned and did. The story I constructed about myself as a biohacker was that I was on a quest of scientific discovery—a quest that felt like a calling for me to embrace a new identity. I wasn't particularly proud of the old story I had been living, and it certainly wasn't helping me recover.

You can either choose to step into your power and embrace this call to adventure, or you can choose not to. That is your choice. You can stay in the victim role as long as you desire—forever if you want. But I know you won't. You already feel the call for something more.

You are being pulled toward your destiny. You believe there's a hero inside you, and you're ready. You may not feel like it yet, but you are fully capable. I guarantee that if you choose the hero's path, help will be readily available along the way. Supernatural aid is always there for the protagonist in mythological stories. The hero is not alone on their journey.

This challenge is an opportunity for you to realize all that you truly are. You're the protagonist of your own inspirational story. You are an explorer, a pioneer, a biohacker. Even if you stop at this step, you will have already made a major change. When you choose a new story, there's a transformation that happens inside you. It's the most important decision you can make.

Triumph is not about winning a war. Triumph is about becoming a warrior. When you set the intention for personal triumph, it brings meaning to your journey. Then you know you were intended to walk this path. This is not something happening to you; it's part of your destiny. You are meant for great things. You decide the narrative. It's time to see yourself as the hero.

7

H: HEED INTUITION

"Be faithful to that which exists nowhere but in yourself."

—André Gide

Now that you've hacked your story and visualized yourself setting out into unknown territory, it's time to learn how to pick your path. You want to have confidence in your treatment decisions. Based on your investigation, you can see many paths you could take. How do you know which is best? What about all the things your doctor or team recommends? You can't do everything, and you certainly can't do it all at once. So how do you prioritize?

The way forward will become clear, but it may not unfold like you expect. In the previous chapters, we talked about thinking of yourself differently and learning new information. In this chapter, we're going to do the opposite. You are going to get out of your head. You're going to enter into the realm of sensing. That is the way to make your health decisions. It's not through thinking that you'll get this knowledge. In fact, your rational brain may even lead you astray.

Thinking out major decisions only works to a point. You can make lists of pros and cons, but that level of thought takes place in your conscious brain. It doesn't get to your deepest level. It doesn't take into account the whole situation, which includes your feelings. What you want when you make an important choice is peace of mind. You want a clear picture of what's best for you.

Unfortunately, thoughts keep bouncing around all the time. That's why the brain can only help so much with decision-making. Eventually, you're just confused and paralyzed in trying to make the "right" choice. Your thinking brain wants to keep weighing options, and you get stuck.

More information isn't what you need to make treatment decisions. Once you have adequately informed yourself, it's time to get out of your head. What you really want is wisdom. Wisdom is all about the heart and gut. When we tap into our other senses, we receive wisdom.

Are you surprised to hear me say that? I may be a biohacker who has studied the brain and likes learning science, but I don't make decisions with my head, and neither should you. Especially when it comes to something as important as your treatment and health. All the information in the world isn't the answer to wisdom. Inner knowing happens on a deeper level.

In school, you were taught to think intellectually rather than to feel. Traditional education prizes rational thought, especially in western society. Someone who can reason out a problem is considered smart. But is that always true? Is it possible to "feel" out a problem instead?

You might be surprised to hear that Albert Einstein's best ideas came when he was shaving his face. He wasn't thinking out solutions. They came to him when he wasn't using reasoning or logic. He got an answer when he did something else. That is how intuition works: we stop relying on our conscious brains and answers just come to us. We get an intuitive "hit."

Einstein believed in intuition. He once said that sometimes he was sure he was right but not sure why. Intuition is when you have a sense about something but you don't know how you know. For example, when you say you have a "hunch" about something—that is your intuition. It is not rational, linear, or fact-based. It is often described as a "gut feeling." It may or may not show up in your abdomen, but the important point is that it's a *sense* of knowing. It's not a thought.

What does intuition feel like? Well, you already know what it's like to have a gut feeling. It's that uneasy feeling you get in the pit of your stomach when you sense you're in danger. Somehow you know that something negative is going to happen. Your body tells you.

Another example is when you have a timely conversation or a significant dream. You might have an "aha" moment when you're talking to a friend, or you may wake up with an insight. It happens when you're least expecting it. The sudden realization brings relief and clarity.

Intuition is sometimes called the sixth sense. Just like your ability to see, hear, smell, taste, and touch, you have this sensory power. It's a valuable resource for biohacking because it's totally individual to you. The information it gives you comes directly from your body. And like a muscle, it gets stronger with use. The more you use your intuition, the better attuned to it you become.

So how do you access your intuition? Well, first you have to be able to recognize it when it shows up. Intuition can show up in various ways, and it's different for every person. You are a unique individual and will learn how it shows up strongest for you. But the most common ways are through your body, dreams, and through signs and synchronicities in the outer world.

Let's start with the body. How does the body communicate information to you? One way is through your instincts. When you have an instinct about something, it means you have a strong inner feeling. It is often your initial reaction to a situation before your analytical mind kicks in. Instincts are highly accurate, which is why they are critical to taking care of your health.

You probably trained yourself to ignore your instincts during the time you went undiagnosed for Lyme. If you're like me, you lost track of the number of times doctors told you your symptoms were all in your head.

You may also have family members who don't believe you because you don't look sick. You've come to doubt and ignore your instincts.

Not trusting that feeling inside when you have a strong instinct about a situation can have dangerous consequences. I nearly lost my life when I ignored signs from my body in favor of listening to my doctors. At the time, I trusted their judgment far more than I trusted my self-knowledge. Rather than listen to my instinct, I talked myself out of seeking immediate medical attention and lost part of my intestines due to a ruptured appendix.

No matter what kind of doctors you're working with, never forget that your instincts are given to you for a reason. They are a part of the innate wisdom you've inherited from our evolutionary history. They are a gift. When you have an instinct, trust it and heed it. Don't let anyone discount it. Above all, don't let your "rational" voice of self-doubt override it.

Our bodies have an awareness of things our minds don't. How can we biohackers use this to our advantage when making treatment and health decisions? One way is through testing the physiology of the body. Traditional doctors often use medical imaging and laboratory tests to see what's going on. They rely on a scan or markers in the blood, stool, urine, saliva, or breath.

This information can be helpful, but it's not a complete picture of what all is going on inside the body. Your body is a complex, energetic system with many stimuli affecting it at once. It's impacted by physical, chemical, electromagnetic, mental, emotional, and spiritual factors.

Even though we are not consciously aware of all that is going on inside us, our nervous system is. As biohackers, we want to be able to tap into this amazing intelligence at work.

You can actually look to the body itself for feedback. Muscle testing is one way to assess the physiology of the body. Your body can indicate whether it is strengthened or weakened by different stimuli and substances. It can actually communicate its needs this way.

How does this work? If you've never experienced muscle testing, it can sound really bizarre. Conventionally trained doctors generally don't use this approach. My introduction to muscle testing was actually in working with a chiropractor long before I tested positive for Lyme. The chiropractor didn't explain what he was up to, and I was convinced he was doing some kind of magic.

As I sat on the examining table, he asked me to hold my arm straight out, parallel to the floor. He repeatedly pressed lightly on it and told me to keep it "strong." Then he proceeded to give me a sequence of small vials to hold in my other hand. With each new vial, he would press on my arm again. It surprised me that there were times I couldn't hold the straight arm up.

It wasn't until he finished that I learned he was testing for allergies to the substances in the vials. He said that when my body was stressed by what was in the vial, my arm went "weak." I thought this method was positively nuts at the time, but years later, I saw the value of this approach. My body had its own language; it could tell me what it didn't want.

Autonomic response testing (ART), developed by Dr. Dietrich Klinghardt, MD, is a more refined method of muscle testing. The autonomic nervous system controls the unconscious bodily functions that are happening all the time. It reacts to stressful stimuli by activating the fight/flight/freeze mode of operation. It's like an internal alarm system. As a result, the stressor blocks proper signaling in the body, and the healing state that is desired is compromised.

How is this useful for making treatment decisions? Well, the treatments that work for one person may not be what another person needs. By testing the body directly, you can get answers that might not show up on a standardized medical test. Muscle testing can identify hidden problems and help you prioritize your treatments based on the findings. It can also indicate whether certain supplements, medications, and other interventions are appropriate for you specifically.

ART and muscle testing help tap into the body's unconscious intelligence. They look directly to the body for guidance rather than to objective laboratory measures or scans. They are also different from relying on a doctor's subjective judgment. Instead, the body is the "expert."

Muscle testing proves that your body is a trustworthy source of information and that it can give you essential feedback as you make decisions about your treatment. Although there are amazing technological advances in the world of biohacking, nothing can match your body's intelligence.

Being a scientist means being open to all creative possibilities for problem-solving. Using intuition is one way to solve a problem or get insight when your analytical brain becomes stuck. When it comes to choosing what is right for your healing, your body is a valuable resource.

When you have an instinctual feeling or get answers through muscle testing, the most important thing you can do is listen. By tuning in to that information rather than tuning it out, you are opening up to receive the direction you desire. Trust that it will come when you ask.

The next step is to acknowledge the messages you get and start putting them into action. As your body tells you what needs attention, have faith that you're getting those messages for a reason. You can now move forward knowing you've got clarity, which brings a sense of inner peace.

8

A: ACT RADICALLY

"In order to carry a positive action we must develop here a positive vision."

—Dalai Lama

Once you've tapped into your intuition for guidance, it's time to take action. Are you ready? I believe you are. This is when the adventure begins. This is when you start seeing results. There is no greater force in the universe than a person's intentional actions. In this chapter, we're going to talk about what that force looks like for your health.

What does it mean to act radically? In this case, I am not talking about "radical" in the sense of something extreme. Here, I mean actions that deal with the "root," or underlying cause. When you do something radical, it doesn't have to be drastic. It can be something small.

What matters is that your actions have a clear purpose that is foundational to your health.

This is the step that distinguishes a biohacker from the typical patient in conventional medicine. Rather than sit back and let your fate be in the doctors' hands, you realize you can take your health into your own hands. It's in the "doing" that the energy of change happens.

You can say, "I want to survive this. I want to get better," but what really indicates your commitment to your healing is what you *do*, not what you say. What you do demonstrates your willingness to truly commit. Without action, you aren't going to get past wishing for recovery.

The most important thing you can realize here is that every positive action step you take matters. This is what will change the whole trajectory of your journey to recovery. It's the major difference between the process of biohacking and mainstream medicine: acting on your own behalf.

When you have a sense of agency in your life, it has a positive effect. Agency is what I describe as having a measure of control and feeling like you can make a difference in the outcome of something. When you take ownership of your health, your body is going to respond accordingly.

This is what's called the "belief effect," or "placebo effect," in traditional medicine. The placebo effect has a negative connotation, but it's actually an amazing phenomenon. Saying that something is a placebo doesn't mean the effect isn't real. The results are a totally valid outcome. What the placebo effect shows is that acting on what we believe can have a positive benefit.

In research, scientists monitor what happens when they give one group an intervention but don't give that intervention to another group. For example, say they're going to test a certain medication. One group in the study receives the medication. The other group unknowingly receives a sham pill, thinking it contains the medication. That is the placebo.

The scientists evaluate the outcome of the study based on who has a positive response to the medication versus the sham pill. The placebo effect is when some participants report a positive response to the sham pill as if they received the medication.

What this tells us is that the very *act* of swallowing a pill can cause a positive outcome. How is that possible? If the sham group didn't take the medication, how could they benefit? It turns out that believing you are going to benefit from something matters.

How is this relevant to your recovery? When you act with the expectation that what you do is going to help you recover, your body benefits physiologically and energetically. The cells in your body and immune system are constantly responding to the internal thought field you generate. You can hack this by setting an intention for your treatments with positive affirmations.

Intention is the power behind manifesting what we desire. But it's not just intending for something to happen, it's putting it into action that sets it into motion. That's why putting money, time, or physical effort toward a goal helps you reach it. You affirm its value and invest in the outcome.

In science, there is something equally as powerful as the placebo effect. It's called the "nocebo effect." This is what happens when a person has a negative expectation rather than a positive one. The opposite outcome is seen with the nocebo effect; the intervention doesn't work or has negative results.

How is the nocebo effect relevant to your recovery? Well, when you engage in something you don't really believe in, your body doesn't get on board. If you're prescribed a treatment protocol from a doctor but don't feel committed to it, it's not going to work.

Is it possible you've had a negative expectation about some of the treatments you've undergone? When you think that something isn't going to work or don't feel a wholehearted belief in what you're doing, the nocebo effect can result in a treatment "failure."

On the other hand, if you view your treatments with a positive mindset—believing that they will be effective— you set an expectation for success. You're proclaiming that you *can* get well. You're setting the intention to live and thrive. This is how you can hack the placebo effect.

In taking action, you can actually reverse engineer your limiting beliefs. For example, if you think you lack self-discipline with food, you can practice intermittent fasting as a way to prove you are disciplined. Doing the thing you think you cannot do works to disprove the limiting belief. When we change our self-perception, we see how powerful we are.

So, where do you start when it comes to taking radical action for your health? How do you know what the "right" thing to do is? That's where your intuition comes into play. The right action is what you feel needs your attention most. You may become aware of the step you need to take through muscle testing, tuning in to your body, or getting insight another way.

People often get stuck in paralysis by analysis, worrying that they will do the wrong thing. They overanalyze to such an extent that they don't take any action. You may find this with treatment protocols and dietary decisions. You think you have to do it all perfectly. The truth is that doing *something* is better than doing *nothing* when it comes to changing your circumstances.

This was one of the most important biohacking lessons in my recovery. Since my doctors were out of state and I lived alone most of the time, I was biohacking everything on my own. When my body was overloaded from the die-off, my pain levels would skyrocket and I would have horrible brain fog. Since the toxicity made it hard to think, I kept a written list of actions to take for detoxification.

I brainstormed all the activities I could do to support circulation and elimination as well as what remedies I could take for drainage. There were so many possibilities: enemas, colonics, sauna therapy, rebounding, dry brushing, lymphatic massage, detox and foot baths, castor-oil packs, PEMF therapy, whole-body vibration, massage, neural therapy, homeopathic remedies, and herbal tinctures. I even made a colorful mindmap on poster board since I'm a visual person.

Whenever I would feel terrible during a Herxheimer reaction and have no idea what to do, I would just pick something and go with it. I trusted that whatever I felt pulled toward was the best action at the time. Sometimes I did several things simultaneously. If I got stuck in thought paralysis, I would close my eyes and put a finger on the page. It was like blindly throwing a dart.

The most important part of dealing with the situation wasn't *what* I did; it was that I did *something*. Doing nothing wasn't going to help my body or mind. If I sat around thinking about how awful I felt, it reinforced how awful I felt. But the minute I picked an action item and followed through on it, I became the director of my experience rather than a spectator.

Biohacking is all about accepting personal responsibility for what you can control. As a biohacker, you are going to start taking action steps, no matter how small, every single day and every single week. That's how you shift the energy to being an agent who's empowered to make a difference in your life.

There are many variables affecting your health that you can take action on. You have control over your lifestyle and behaviors. You can hack your home or work environment. You can create new, healthy habits.

That is how you have the power to change your inner biology.

The habits that affect our health include what we put in our mouth, what we put on our body, our sleep "hygiene," our exposure to sunlight and blue light, our movement, our thinking patterns, our social connections, and our exposure to electromagnetic radiation and environmental factors, such as mold, and other toxins, like chemicals, heavy metals, pesticides, unhealthy air, etc.

When it comes to taking action, you can start by creating habits. The key is repetition. What you do every day is what creates big changes. Start with what you put in your mouth and on your body, then look at what you listen to, read, and watch. Only you can set boundaries around what goes into your body and mind. You can biohack your inner and outer environment.

Acting radically is about taking back control of your biology and doing whatever it takes to get to the root causes of your health problems. It's about addressing all levels of well-being, including physiological, mental, emotional, energetic and even spiritual. When you have a protocol you believe in and you take action on it every day, you create momentum toward your vision.

9

C: CONQUER FEAR

"Inaction breeds doubt and fear. Action breeds confidence and courage. If you want to conquer fear, do not sit home and think about it. Go out and get busy."

—Dale Carnegie

I've just finished telling you how taking action and targeting root causes are the most important principles of biohacking. When it comes to treating Lyme and improving your health, so much of it is dependent on your ability to step up, design action steps, and follow through on those action steps.

So the next question becomes "What happens if I can't take action? What happens if I'm too afraid of doing something new? What happens if I feel anxious about what might happen? What if I feel like I can't move forward?" That's what we're going to address in this chapter.

Our brains are designed to go into protective mode whenever they perceive we're in danger. The nervous system stays alert, looking for threats. It looks for what could go wrong in any situation, even when there is no real danger. Our brains will imagine that something is a threat even if it isn't. Then we become consumed by thoughts that slow us down or stop us in our tracks.

Picture a young child who sees shadows in the dark. The shadows look like a monster or some other figment of the child's imagination. Does that mean there is actually a monster just because the child believes it to be so? No. It's just the brain's protection system in overdrive.

Our brains have an amazing capacity for imagination. It's one of our greatest assets; it's what makes us creatures who can innovate and evolve. We imagine possible scenarios and then prepare ourselves to react appropriately to situations we haven't experienced before.

But can our brains go too far and cause us to react unnecessarily? Absolutely. Just like the child who sees those shadows and imagines a monster. The monster appears to be real, but that doesn't mean the shadows are actually something to be afraid of.

The part of the brain that is constantly trying to protect us is called the limbic system. It contains a structure called the amygdala, which processes emotions. When something causes us anxiety, the amygdala triggers a fight/flight/freeze response. This reactivity was quite helpful in our evolutionary history. But these days it's a little more complicated than that.

The limbic brain is what allowed ancient human beings to survive in environments where there was danger. It kept them safe by allowing them to prepare for potential threats and react accordingly when those threats were real. Thanks to the amygdala, human beings survived in environments with predators by using emotions like fear to their advantage.

But the limbic brain isn't always helpful when we're afraid or anxious. It tends to go into overdrive when it can't make sense of a situation. Because its job is to protect us, it constructs scenarios about any potential harm we might be facing. It comes up with all sorts of possibilities.

What happens when the fight/flight/freeze mechanism kicks in unnecessarily? We become paralyzed by thinking of potential outcomes that may never happen. An acronym I love is FEAR: false evidence appearing real. Even though the threat seems real to us, it's not based on truth, it's based on false evidence. It's based on the story we're constructing about the evidence.

So, when it comes to taking action, what kind of threats is your brain is projecting? Your brain will come up with lots of reasons as to why you shouldn't do something you haven't done before or change an old behavior. The limbic system stores memories and wants to draw from those memories to keep you safe. Anything new or different is a threat.

With any treatment or health intervention, your brain will put the brakes on you by asking, "What if the outcome isn't what I want? What if I hurt myself? What if it doesn't work? What if other people don't approve? What if the problem gets worse? What if I can't follow through?"

Doing something we've never done seems scary because we've never done it, but the only way we can stop being afraid of something we fear is to do it. There's no other way to get past it. You get past fear by moving through it, not going around it.

So just how do we do this? First, we actually have to appreciate the fear for what it is. You can acknowledge why it cropped up: it was trying to protect you. But you can assure your limbic system that you don't need protection from everything new or different. You can think back to experiences where you did something for the first time and things were okay.

You have to learn how to act in spite of fear because you really can't "outthink" fear. You're never going to conquer your fears by thinking about them. What works to conquer a fear is action. Even though the fear may crop up, the goal is to continue forward with the action.

When I first started biohacking, I experienced a lot of fear whenever I tried new treatments, especially if those treatments were things I investigated on my own and not prescribed by my doctors. I'm grateful my brain kicked in with a healthy fear response because it gave me a reason to become fully informed and proceed cautiously. I did my homework and prepared myself.

Once I learned about the science behind a new therapy, I would feel more optimistic. Instead of thinking about what could go wrong, I focused on what could go right. I got more excited. I was seeing all the possibilities for good. If I had spent time imagining all the worst-case scenarios, I would never have tried many of the treatments that worked for me.

Even when I could see that there was nothing rational about my fears, that didn't stop them from arising. I came to realize that trying to talk myself out of them was pointless. My brain was just doing its job, and I could appreciate that. But I could talk myself into acting anyway.

When you decide to act in spite of your fear, you shut down the power it has over you. It's doing the very thing you're afraid of that puts you back in a place of personal power. You prove you can do whatever you put your mind to. You find courage within yourself.

This means sometimes choosing to take on a new "identity." It means acting as if you aren't afraid. Have you ever heard the phrase "Fake it until you make it"? That's what I'm talking about here. You can't wait to feel courageous. You have to fake it until you feel it.

Visualization is a powerful tool for overcoming your fears. Seeing yourself doing the thing you feel afraid of helps your brain "experience" you doing it for the first time. Your brain doesn't know the difference between the visualization and the actual act. This gets the brain used to the idea of something new. You can practice by imagining yourself doing it successfully.

Fears are like dragons along your journey. As the hero, you have to confront them to continue on your path. If you don't slay the dragons in your way, you can't move forward. You can think of the dragon as guarding a valuable treasure: a better state of health. Don't let fear keep you from the treasure. You can slay any dragon. The courage will come as you act.

I never imagined myself being able to do the things I've done to get well over the years: administering my own intravenous treatments, daily neural therapy and intramuscular injections, intermittent and extended fasting, experimenting with do-it-yourself treatments— and going against the advice of mainstream doctors and dieticians. As you go along your own journey, you too will discover the strength to do what you need to.

Whenever you feel fear, think of it as an opportunity for growth, a chance to expand beyond the belief that you *can't*. You will prove to yourself that you *can*. As a biohacker, you will realize how powerful you really are. With each action you take, you will realize that fear is a construct of the mind. When you free your mind from limitation, you free your body as well.

10

K: KNOCK DOWN OBSTACLES

"We are all faced with a series of great opportunities brilliantly disguised as insoluble problems."

—John W. Gardner

All right, let's move on to the next step. Now you know that fear is not going to stop you; in fact, it's your very fear you're going to take action on. But you are still going to encounter other obstacles. Your job on this journey is to knock down every obstacle you come to. In this chapter, we're going to talk about how the biohacker addresses obstacles.

The first thing to know is that obstacles are going to arise no matter what. But remember that you have a choice about your mindset. You can choose to think of yourself as a victim in these circumstances or as a hero. Obstacles aren't happening to you; they just happen. They are a fact of life.

But you choose how you approach each obstacle; you can use them as an opportunity to grow and use creative problem-solving, or you can let them defeat you. If you see each obstacle as part of your greater destiny, you know it was given to you as a challenge to overcome.

Remember what it felt like to envision yourself as the hero? Being the hero means having a strong will. That is what can get you through these challenges: having the will to make it through. This path that you're taking is not an easy one. But where there is a will, there is always a way.

Your confidence will grow as you knock down the obstacles along the way. You'll begin feeling better about yourself than you've ever felt in your whole life. You'll actually feel like a superhero. You will be filled with a sense of inner strength and faith that you can get through anything.

The second thing to know is that the obstacles are going to suck. I'm not going to sugarcoat it; you're well aware of how difficult it is to go through this journey of recovery. Even if the challenges help you grow and teach you positive life lessons, they can still absolutely suck.

To recover from Lyme, I had to learn "embrace the suck" because it was what I had to go through to get better. What was difficult in the short run was helping me in the long run. Bodybuilders or athletes say short-term pain leads to long-term gain. In biohacking, the principle of hormesis describes how an organism can benefit from biological adaptations to stressors.

As you overcome the obstacles of your journey, you become stronger and more resilient. You become more adapted for future challenges. You'll know you're capable of getting through them too because you've gotten through Lyme disease. With each challenge we overcome, we increase our capacity. Our goal is to become the best individual we can be.

Some of the obstacles you may face will be physically painful. You might need to undergo various surgeries if you have cavitations in the jawbone, teeth with root-canal fillings, chronically infected tonsils, breast implants, or metal implants in your body. Recovering from these surgeries is painful—there's no doubt about it. But these can be the root causes of illness.

As a biohacker, you are going to tackle these obstacles with the knowledge that eliminating hidden sites of infection will unburden your immune system from pathogens and toxicity. Realize that you won't necessarily know of hidden infections just because there's no pain or inflammation at the site.

For example, you may not have a sore throat despite chronic tonsillitis, or breast tenderness if you have implants. There may be no localized symptoms of infection. However, there's an overall burden on the immune system from too many pathogens. It's like an army fighting a war on many fronts.

Pathogens can remain protected from your immune cells when they are surrounded by biofilm or live in areas that don't get good blood flow, like the jawbone.

Even though there may be no outward signs of infection, the pathogens release toxins.

The body is a complex electrical system within which everything is connected. A problem in one place in the body can affect many distant locations. For example, each tooth is connected to other bodily systems, so you may have symptoms elsewhere that appear unrelated. This is how periodontal disease links to heart disease.

Traditional medicine would focus on treating symptoms where they are detected. When doctors diagnose heart disease, they typically prescribe medication. But what if the root cause is gum disease? Biohacking means looking underneath the presenting symptoms to find the source of the problem. Fixing the problem will allow the body to heal, and the symptoms will go away. That's the goal of these interventions.

These obstacles to your healing need to be knocked down. There may be no indication that there is a problem using basic x-ray imaging; more specific types of imaging are necessary. Muscle testing and specific laboratory tests can show what your individual needs may be.

These are obstacles you can prepare for in advance. Planning for a surgery allows you to brainstorm strategies for how you will support your body afterward. You can order supplements, schedule intravenous therapy, make bodywork appointments, and learn biohacking techniques. Forethought helps you get in the right mindset and get practical strategies in place.

Other obstacles in your path will be things you can't prepare for until they happen. They are like getting hit by lightning. These types of obstacles will tempt you to lapse into feeling like a victim—if you let them. It's with these challenges that you have to find your inner hero.

Even though it may feel like circumstances are out of your control, the one thing you can control is your mindset. You can choose how you see the situation and how you respond to it. You either accept that it has happened and rise to the challenge, or you let it overtake you.

You can make it through anything you are facing. It may take every ounce of courage and strength to get through it, but I promise you can. There is nothing you can't overcome. Even when you go through hell and it seems like it will never end, know that it too shall pass.

My recovery from unexpected intestinal surgery was the hardest thing I've ever done. But I gained so much in the process: I found out I was courageous enough to defy the doctors in the hospital despite their intimidation, I learned to do my own intravenous injections, and realized I needed to keep doing monthly parasite treatment around the full moon and new moon.

All the obstacles I faced on my journey taught me there's a reason for everything that shows up in life. There is the potential for good to come out of any situation. After I was in a head-on car accident during a very dark time in my life, my physical therapy probably saved me from suicide. It reminded me that I needed to be strong in my body and renewed my determination to get well.

Having gratitude is so difficult amid hardship. When it feels like things can't get any worse, it takes a lot of work to think of what you're grateful for. Writing it down or telling someone else helps. Whenever you feel gratitude, you are hacking the mind and body state.

Your mindset is especially important when it comes to getting your hands on resources, technologies, and health-related supplies. You are going to encounter obstacles because of FDA restrictions and Big Pharma's efforts to limit what's available directly to consumers. Solutions that are effective for improving health and reversing chronic disease are a threat to their profits.

Being committed to the process of biohacking means you get creative and resourceful. Where you might have formerly relied on prescriptions and things to be given to you by doctors, you're now going to be a pioneer. It's going to take some effort.

But the good news is that you can crowdsource with other biohackers and that you'll benefit collectively. As a biohacking community, we can share what we are learning and where to get resources. Many consumer products and even medications can be ordered from overseas suppliers, and there is now laboratory testing you can order for yourself in the United States.

It will take innovation and creativity for you to knock down some of the obstacles. I have used compounding pharmacies all over the world to obtain certain medications. Since the laws in the United States vary by state as to what they can dispense and where they can ship, you have to do your homework. Many veterinary sources for parasite treatment can be accessed directly online.

When you choose to look at every challenge as an opportunity for innovation, your mind opens up to what the solutions can be. Remember that a biohacker doesn't look at what's been done before; a biohacker says, "How do I discover a new solution to this problem?"

It is about being playful even in the face of an obstacle. When you think outside the box, you will start to resource your own creativity. You will join forces with other creative individuals and grow together. What was once a challenge will lead to new discoveries.

The most important thing you can decide for yourself is that you're not going to take no for an answer. When you hit an obstacle in your path, know that it's an opportunity to find another way. It's not a roadblock unless you let it stop you. There is always a way forward.

11

E: EXPERIMENT WISELY

"A person who never made a mistake never tried anything new."

—Albert Einstein

So you're prepared to knock down obstacles and take action in spite of fear. The next thing we need to address is how you go about experimenting as a biohacker. This is where the adventure becomes exhilarating. Your body becomes your test ground, and new insights await.

Scientific work is based on observation and reproducing results through experimentation. The scientific method involves making hypotheses and observing experimental findings. Biohacking uses this method but on a smaller scale. You are the only subject in the experiment. In science, we represent the people in a study as the number n; so as a biohacker, you are $n = 1$.

How is biohacking different than following a standardized protocol for Lyme treatment? It is this process of self-experimentation. You're learning what else is out there and trying it for yourself. As a biohacker, you are not like the typical Lyme patient waiting to be told what to do. You know your health is in your hands and there are infinite possibilities you want to explore.

So what does it look like to experiment on your own? Biohacking does not mean being foolhardy or reckless. How can you try out treatments or therapies on yourself in a wise manner?

Good scientists use critical thinking skills and are methodical in their approach. They collect data and pay attention to details. They gather unbiased information and do their research in advance.

It's important to remember that scientists are also courageous and visionary thinkers. They think outside the box and entertain revolutionary ideas. Their discoveries may challenge accepted theories. Good scientists try what has never been tried and learn from their mistakes.

Let's talk a little about making mistakes. It's common to become overly concerned with making mistakes when you start biohacking. There's a learning curve, and making mistakes is part of that learning curve. Things are not going to go perfectly on the first try. That's not realistic.

What you have to keep in mind is that medicine is really just a practice in conducting experiments. When a doctor puts you on a treatment protocol, it's a process of experimentation. Doctors hypothesize about what might work to treat your conditions, gather information from testing, decide on a plan of action, and then observe results.

So, as a biohacker, you're going to be following the same process. That's not to say you're being your own doctor. Remember that you have a team and are working with different kinds of doctors and people providing ideas, information, and resources to help you.

Biohacking is simply adopting the scientific method of thinking. It's what doctors use to come up with solutions for their patients, or at least, that's what they're supposed to do. However, as we've already discussed, many doctors aren't good scientists. They are just thinking about symptom treatment instead of the root causes of health problems.

Good doctors try to assess the underlying causes of disease and prescribe what they think will work to correct the situation. But even with the best analysis and testing, they can't know for sure what will work. To a certain extent, the practice of medicine is just that—a practice, a process of trial and error.

Doctors make mistakes all the time. Even the treatments your doctor prescribes can cause unforeseen consequences and seriously harm you. Hospitalizations and deaths from prescribed medications and drug interactions are extremely common. Just because a doctor puts you on a treatment doesn't mean they can predict the outcome. They are making calculated guesses.

There were a lot of mistakes made during my recovery. Even with the best doctors and regular ART testing, I often had unpredictable reactions. Several different treatments I underwent resulted in my having seizures because there was so much die-off in my brain. I had allergic reactions to certain injections that scarred my skin. And immunotherapy dosing wasn't always reliable, even with ART.

It's not that my doctors were doing anything unsafe, they were just doing what doctors and scientists do. They try things and hope for the best with as much testing and research as they can gather beforehand. The reality is that every patient is a test subject and there are always unintended mishaps or unforeseen consequences. How a person is going to react is an unknown.

What I learned is that you just have to deal with mistakes and move on. Some mishaps are bigger than others, of course. My seizures landed me in the hospital more than once. When my doctors miscommunicated with each other before one surgery, I contracted a life-threatening infection and had to be hospitalized. When the doses of my immunotherapy were too high, I would Herx badly.

Of course, I've made plenty of mistakes myself. I've overdosed on my own treatment and had to spend days doing extra detox. I've pushed the time limits for having a chest port and PICC line because I wanted to continue my home IV therapy. I've spent many sleepless nights taking baths and doing colonics and neurofeedback to deal with toxicity and brain inflammation.

I had to learn to deal with the fallout, both from my own experiments and from doctor-prescribed treatments. That meant a lot of self-care and bodywork to clean up the messes. But the human body is amazingly resilient. It took time and effort, but my body recovered.

Biohacking technologies can help the body heal and recover faster from toxic overload, injury, and stress. Pulsed electromagnetic field (PEMF) and red-light therapies can help the body detoxify faster, reducing pain and inflammation. These also stimulate mitochondrial function and boost your body's voltage, which is key to healing. You need enough voltage to make new cells.

Scientists can't know how experiments are going to go before they run them. They simply observe the outcome and figure out what to do differently the next time. If they want to reproduce the result, they do it the same way again. If they want a different result, they change it.

As a biohacker, your mindset needs to be that mistakes are just feedback. The results you get help you modify the experimental design for next time. Even mistakes yield information and allow you to learn from what you did. You're constantly evaluating as you go along. You make observations and track the results based on the variable you change each time.

Even if you don't realize it, you already have experience as a biohacker. You've been monitoring your symptoms in order to report back to your doctor. With biohacking, you're going to become more scientific about following your progress with each health intervention.

Using a notebook or a calendar is key to remembering what you do. Brain fog makes it hard to keep it all straight unless you write it down. As you try treatments, supplements, or therapies, you want to record the following: What was the dose? What was the outcome? What changed in your symptoms? What improvements are you seeing? Is anything getting worse?

Assessing your progress can be done with subjective observations or quantifiable measurements. It's valuable to use a logbook or spreadsheet to monitor your bloodwork, heavy-metal levels, and other variables as they change over time. It will be motivating when you see success. There are many biohacking technologies and apps that will track data for you as well.

Only you can decide what is worth experimenting with. If something muscle tests positively for your body, then your body is saying yes to that intervention. When your intuition guides you to something, you can trust that as well. Ultimately, you are the lead decision-maker.

To improve my health, I have tried just about every treatment strategy imaginable. There was nothing I wouldn't do to get well. The more strategies I tried, the more I could see the possibility of recovery. And when I saw positive results, I got excited. I felt like a pioneer charting new territory.

I learned how to carefully increase my dosages to see what I could tolerate. When I wasn't seeing results anymore, I'd increase the dose. If I got a Herxheimer reaction, I'd decrease it slightly and increase my drainage and detoxification. The same thing was true when I used

Rife frequencies. If I could tolerate a certain intensity, I would increase the level during the next session.

It's important to realize that dosing is key to any treatment for Lyme, co-infections, and viral or fungal infections. Any treatment that is given at too high of a dose can cause a Herxheimer reaction. In fact, any substance administered to the body in excess can be toxic, including water. Many substances are therapeutic in small amounts but dangerous in large doses.

The key to experimenting wisely on yourself is getting accurate information beforehand, starting at a very low dose (or duration), and monitoring your body's reactions. You also need to check for any potential interactions with the other items in your protocol. Muscle testing can be useful for knowing how stressed the body is and when to take a break or back down on the dose.

Experimenting wisely is necessary so you don't overdo anything. You want your treatments to be effective without putting your body under too much stress at once. As you decrease the pathogen load and cleanse any toxicity, your body will be able to tolerate more. At that point, the positive results of your biohacking experimentation will be something to celebrate!

12

R: RISK BRAVELY

"Take calculated risks. Act boldly and thoughtfully."

—Ray Kroc

Experimenting wisely is how you discover for yourself what improves your health. The more you experiment, the more confidence and experience you'll gain. You'll realize you're ready for more. Biohacking is all about reaching your full biological potential. It's about trying things and having new experiences. It's about testing the waters and stepping out of your comfort zone.

When it comes to doing anything new in life, there is a certain degree of risk involved. Biohacking is no different. Being a biohacker involves risk because you don't know how your experiments will turn out. You have to accept the uncertainty of the outcome before you act. It may not turn out the way you want, but if you don't try, you'll never know.

So my question for you is: How big is your brave?

I know some of you will think you're not brave enough to go this route. You might think the risks associated with biohacking are too great. But what do you have to lose? Isn't the greatest risk staying where you are? Isn't the greatest risk continuing to do what you've been doing? If your goal is to get somewhere new, you're never going to do that by treading the same path.

In gambling, people take risks all the time, right? They throw money into a game whether or not they expect to win. They're hoping for a good outcome. But not all gamblers are being foolish when they risk their money. How do they decide what to bet on?

Gambling involves using one's intuition, or gut feeling. It's about having a hunch about what to put a bet on, not knowing what's going to happen. Sure, people can look at the odds and statistics, but in the end, they're basically hoping and praying for the result they want.

The process of biohacking isn't so much like gambling as it is like making a long-term financial investment in which you expect a positive reward. That's what you do when you invest; you make a commitment believing it's going to yield financial gain.

In investing, risk typically equals reward. When you risk a nominal amount, usually you expect that the return is also going to be a nominal amount. For example, if you put a quarter into a slot machine, you don't expect to win $10,000.

But what happens when you risk a lot more? There's the possibility of a much greater payout. When you make a large investment in something, you expect a greater reward. Biohacking is kind of like that. The biohacker is saying, "I expect that my actions are going to pay off. I have faith that what I'm doing will benefit my health."

Of course, I am not talking about blind risk-taking here. As a biohacker, you want to be well-informed, do your homework, consult with more-experienced people, start things cautiously, and monitor yourself closely. You also must ensure that nothing you do will cause harm to anyone else.

Ultimately, however, all that research and preparation does not guarantee the outcome. There can be no guarantee on how your body will respond to something you've never done. That's the unknown. As a biohacker, when you decide to experiment with something new, you're taking a calculated risk.

What helps you know whether a risk is worth taking? You have to go back to your body's intuition. Only your instinct, or gut feeling, can guide you to what is right for you. As you make treatment decisions and evaluate lifestyle changes, you have to feel it out for yourself.

As I started biohacking, I was nervous about doing anything that might "break the rules." I had never been rebellious in my whole life. But I soon learned that I would need to buck more than just the medical system. In order to be a biohacker, I was going to have to become a rebel.

It was not easy at first. I was nervous all the time. Even though I wasn't breaking any laws, I was constantly questioned. Going through airport security lines, I got flagged by TSA for traveling with medical devices, and even my service dog had to go through additional screening.

They would remove all my biohacking tools from my carry-on bags and thoroughly search all my checked luggage. Apparently, things like an enema bag, plastic tubing, nebulizer, massage tools, dry brushes, canned sardines, and frozen meat were "suspicious" items.

I got used to this kind of treatment over time since I was flying on airplanes frequently. It became normal for people to look at me strangely since I wrapped myself in a blanket of silver fabric for protection from electromagnetic radiation, wore a mask, and preboarded flights with a service dog. Eventually I didn't care.

When I started researching alternative solutions, the risks were greater because of FDA restrictions and the lack of coverage by medical insurance. I had to get very creative to obtain non-FDA approved self-care devices, European health products, certain medications, and IV supplies.

Becoming a biohacker meant stepping out of my old mindset and into a new way of thinking. The old me worried about what other people thought and feared getting caught even when I wasn't doing anything wrong. The new me started to see through my fears and let them go.

How does a person become more risk tolerant? We already talked about how the brain doesn't like to feel threatened. Anything that seems risky is going to automatically send the limbic system into fight/flight/freeze mode. It won't matter if this is a real danger to you or not.

What happens to the body when you think about taking a risk? In short, it gets stressed. Your whole nervous system reacts, activating your body for defense or escape. This evolutionary response actually quickens your pulse and breathing and increases your muscle tension.

What can be done to calm the nervous system? Since the body is physically activated, you need to address the physical level. This will reduce anxiety. Biofeedback techniques, breath work, neurofeedback, massage, and other forms of relaxation therapy all work to calm the stress.

Visualizing yourself taking the risk and having a successful outcome is very important. When you imagine the result you want in advance, your brain gets some relief from the anxiety. You create a positive memory of having already done it. The more you visualize, the better.

Whether you see yourself as brave or not, you can proceed by acting as if you are. Just like conquering any fear, when you take a risk, you act in spite of it. You say, "I am not willing to live in fear." You don't start out feeling brave. You'll feel the bravery kick in as you act.

This means you're going to have to fake it until you make it. One way to boost your confidence is to hack your posture or engage in physical activity. By adjusting your posture, you can actually create a feeling of power in the body. Your body sends the feedback to your brain. I like to straighten my back and put my hands on my hips, like a superhero. Your "power pose" can be anything that works for you. You can also exercise or listen to music to pump you up.

When it comes to risk, there will always be a certain amount of anxiety you will feel about it. That's really okay; it's not a bad thing. It helps you plan adequately for what you want to do. When you're a little bit anxious, you prepare yourself both physically and mentally.

You're not making the decision from a place of fear, however. When your intuition guides you to take a risk, you are trusting the gut feeling that says you're doing the right thing. That sense of inner knowing will be more powerful than the fear. There is a part of you that's unafraid.

Making health decisions involves taking calculated risks. You have to decide what the desired result is worth to you and how much you're willing to gamble or invest in the process. The more bravely you risk, the more you grow comfortable risking.

When I first started on my biohacking journey, my risks were small. I would investigate new treatments but wait to try them. I'd ask my doctor before doing anything. But over time, I started becoming braver. I would try things before I had doctor appointments and give the doctors the results. I'd follow my intuition and adjust my treatment dosing to higher and higher levels.

What I realized was, who dares, wins. I got bigger rewards from bigger risks. Sometimes I would overshoot the dosing and have a Herxheimer reaction, but then I knew the treatment was effective. Ultimately, I decided I'd rather gain my life by risking big than lose my life to Lyme.

There was nothing I wasn't willing to do to get well. There was no treatment I wouldn't try. There was no amount of money, time, energy, or resources I wouldn't devote to healing. I was willing to risk a lot, even if I made mistakes. I would do whatever it took to recover.

It wasn't easy because, over and over again, I had to make the decision that I was worth it. My life was worth fighting for because I deserved to be healthy. That was difficult for me at first. I had been sick for so long I didn't know if that was possible. But I could envision it for myself.

I had to deal with a lot of controversy about my choices. In the beginning, people expressed concern about the risks I was taking. Although I informed my doctors of everything I did, some people thought my protocols, diet, and self-administered treatments were unsafe.

For the most part, I didn't share with other people unless they expressly wanted to learn for their own healing. It's really no one else's business what I do to take care of my health. I trusted my research, my intuition, my team of consultants, and the results of my biohacking.

Your risk tolerance will be different than that of your family or friends. You will need to decide for yourself what kind of boundaries you want to keep. Many people will not understand your choices. They will stay stuck in the old paradigm. Fear is a big factor in that paradigm.

Being brave is about taking a stand against fear. It's about being willing to risk doing what's out of the norm or break the "rules" that violate your freedom. If you were no longer frightened, what risks would you take? What might be possible for you? Who could you be?

You need to know that being brave is not about feeling brave. Being brave is about a choice; it's choosing what you're willing to do for yourself. It is through taking the big leaps that we learn to fly. It is only through trying things we have never done that we see what we can achieve. I know you are brave enough to get well. You are going to prove that to yourself.

Recovering from Lyme is just the start. Biohacking is an adventure in which your health gains will spur you on in other areas of life. The braver you become, the more possibilities open up. The good news is that your future lies ahead of you. This journey will actually set you free.

13

"HOW DO I DO THIS?"

"Our doubts are traitors, and make us lose the good we oft might win, by fearing to attempt."

—William Shakespeare

There you have it. I've laid out for you the basic principles of biohacking in an order that is variable but makes sense: how to begin thinking like a biohacker, how to start making decisions for yourself, how to tune in to your body and receive intuitive guidance, how to take action with confidence, how to deal with setbacks, how to experiment based on your own feedback, how to recalibrate when you encounter unexpected results, and lastly, how to be brave.

You may look back and see that you've been waiting for someone else to come up with the solutions. You may see you haven't fully trusted yourself—your voice, your body, your intuition. You've been waiting for somebody else to provide the answers and heal you from the outside. For so long, you were sure that if you found the right doctor or the right treatment plan, all your problems would be solved. You were waiting for a fairy godmother to wave a magic wand.

Unfortunately, that's just not the way the universe works. It requires us to be participants. It requires our actions. It requires us to be partners with the field of energy. We connect with that energy and get direction. But we get to be the actors and producers of our lives. We get to be agents of our own choosing. That's what's called free will.

Manifestation is not about a magic wand that delivers our wishes; it's about us delivering our own wishes. It's about committing to the creative process. It's about us being on board, being all in. It's about our co-creation with the universe, our co-creation with our team, our co-creation in the field of intention. That's what we can do for our health; that's what biohacking is all about.

Biohacking is a different framework. Biohacking is not about sitting back and waiting for doctors or "experts" to have all the answers. Biohacking is about saying, "Hey, I'm on board. I'm a participant. I'm going to help myself. I'm going to engage with the entire field of potential. I'm going to work with my body. I'm going to use the power of my body to improve my health."

Biohacking is all about moving from belief in limitation to belief in limitless possibilities. It's about proclaiming, "Abundant health is possible. It is possible for me. I believe my body has the power to heal. I believe there is something I can participate in to help it. I want to help my body function optimally so that I can be the best version of myself on this planet."

What does it mean to believe in the "impossible"? Well, the very word breaks down into the words "I'm possible." So, really, it means choosing to believe that something is possible even if you haven't seen evidence of it. Believing in your recovery from Lyme might feel like believing in the impossible. This is where the biohacking mindset becomes necessary. You have to start by proclaiming that health is possible for you, even if you haven't seen it yet.

What comes up for you when you think of taking this different approach? Is there resistance? Is there fear? What about limiting beliefs? Those are the obstacles you're going to encounter when you start to think about becoming a biohacker. Just as with anything else in life, deciding to make some major changes to your treatment approach can be daunting.

Whenever we think about doing something new, our brain has a built-in protection mode. It's like an immune system that guards against us making change. It tries to keep us safe. Except in this case it's not actually helping you; it's keeping you stuck in a cycle of doing what you've always done. Thinking in the old ways is routine; it feels comfortable.

Becoming a biohacker means undertaking a big overhaul in how you think and how you act. It means changing how you see yourself with respect to doctors. It means taking complete ownership of your health and letting go of blame. It means embracing a beginner's mind rather than your ego. It means learning new things that contradict old ideas. It means stopping habits that come from a lifetime of programming and creating new behaviors.

One obstacle you are going to face is internal resistance. Totally changing your personal habits, nutrition, home environment, and relationship dynamics feels overwhelming at first. As a biohacker, you have to be willing to make significant changes to optimize your health.

Changing the way you spend your time and how you eat, move, sleep, and interact with others is something a lot of people don't want to do. It requires taking a hard look at what isn't working for you and eliminating the behaviors, substances, foods, and toxic energy from your life.

Then it requires putting your time, energy, money, and resources toward the things you want to see improve. It can be a lot of work to turn your health around. It takes a daily commitment to make time for self-care, maintaining a healthy home environment and educating yourself.

How willing are you to put time, energy, and money toward yourself? What is it worth to you? Your health is the ultimate act of proclaiming your self-worth. You have to be willing to do the work, and you have to do it on a regular basis. This is a commitment to a new lifestyle.

You will also face external resistance as you change your treatment approach and health habits. Changing your habits can be threatening to the people around you. They might not like the "new" you as you become more empowered as a biohacker. You may face disapproval about your choices or undergo questioning that makes you uncomfortable. This can bring up some fear.

It's scary to do things your doctor, family, or friends disagree with. It might even mean losing friends or partners who don't want to face their own health habits. As soon as you start doing something different, those people don't feel as good about themselves anymore. They don't want to be around this version of you. They may say they liked the "old" you better.

That can certainly happen. And it can be really awkward because you don't want to feel alienated. It's hard to stand up to family or friends who don't respect your autonomy or who question you outright. You might feel like you have to "know it all" to validate your choices. This can bring up feelings of inadequacy or the limiting beliefs you have had since childhood.

Another source of resistance may actually come unknowingly from your loved ones. Although they believe they truly want you to see you healthy, their lives have been influenced by your illness for years. They are used to being in the role of caretaker or provider. They are used to seeing you limited by your current condition and may even treat you like a "victim."

This can reinforce an old mindset for you. It can be hard for them to appreciate the change in mindset you want to make. You may find it hard to not revert to old ways of thinking about yourself.

It's also become "normal" for you to see yourself as ill. You've gotten used to it. Your whole identity has been defined by years of illness. Even if you think you are ready to be well, your subconscious doesn't know how to make sense of that yet. It has adapted to the current reality. To shift to something else is going to throw you for a loop. The subconscious mind won't like it.

It can be helpful to look at any internal resistance to this new approach by asking yourself some questions. What is this illness holding for you? How are you benefiting from staying ill? Is it that you're comfortable and that you don't have to come into your power?

That's what a lot of people are scared of. They're scared of the idea of being healthy. Does that sound crazy? It's not. I know this has been surprisingly true for me. As I got healthier and healthier, it filled me with fear. I had no idea who I was anymore. I'd been sick for so long, that's all I knew.

Stepping out of that paradigm of illness was like stepping out of a cave and into a blinding light. What would be expected of me if I was healthy? It was almost enough for me to turn back around and stay in hibernation. It would've been much more comfortable to keep hiding.

Except something was calling me out of the cave, something I couldn't ignore. It was like I was being pulled toward that blinding light. And it was scary as hell because I knew only darkness. But I felt like a life of illness wasn't supposed to be my ultimate identity.

A lot of people get blocked by fear. For some, it's the fear of making a mistake or not doing things perfectly. For others, it's the fear that biohacking is unpredictable or risky. Still others might be afraid that nothing will work.

But the fears also may not be what you think they are. For a lot of you, the fear is about what happens if things do work. All you know is illness. All you know is pain. You don't even know what your life would be like if you didn't have suffering.

Maybe the fear isn't that you're going to lose your life. Maybe the fear is that you're going to gain your life. Maybe the fear is that you've never let yourself dream big or think big. Maybe you've never believed you are worthy. What might be possible if you did believe you were worthy of abundant health? What might you do with your unlimited, untapped potential?

The very fact that you picked up this book tells me you feel your destiny is calling you. Deep inside, there's a sneaking suspicion that you have the power within you to do great things. If you weren't ready for a change, I promise you wouldn't have lasted this long. The fact that you've made it this far in the book tells me you're ready to step into your power.

If you take on the biohacking mindset, you're proclaiming to the universe, "I am worthy. I am worthy of health and well-being. I am ready to take on a new identity. I am ready to take the next steps. I am committed to loving myself more. I am committed to life. I want to think bigger. I want to be bigger. I want to know my power. I want to see what good I can do in this world."

Does that sound terrifying? I bet it does. It certainly did to me. Stepping out of the darkness into the light was both terrifying and exhilarating. Quite honestly, it still is. Every day that I proclaim myself as a biohacker, I am consciously choosing a new way of being. I am affirming my belief in myself. I'm still working on that; it doesn't come naturally at all.

You are at a crossroads now. You can either choose to claim this new identity for yourself or not. Ultimately, the question is what do you have to lose? You're sick; you're stuck in a rut. Why not change things up? Why not lay it all on the line to see what can happen?

If you adopt the mindset of a biohacker, you're deciding with your actions that you're willing to step out of the old paradigm. You're shifting to a revolutionary way of thinking about your health.

Recovering from illness takes a willingness to be bold and choose your own path. It's an investment of your time, energy, and resources. Fundamentally, it's an investment in yourself. It will not be an easy road, but it will be worth it. It's worth it because you are worth it.

Either you can work your way through these potential speed bumps or you can let them block you from moving forward. What do you see yourself getting blocked by?

Will you get hung up on the difficulty of changing your habits? Will you lapse back into your old story or let other people influence you negatively? Will you lose sight of your vision for the future? Will you doubt your capability and intuition?

As you work through these challenges, you will be transforming yourself and your life. So, are you going to be blocked? Or are you going to step into your power?

14

"WHERE DO I GO FROM HERE?"

"Life expects something of you, and it is up to every individual to discover what it should be."

—Victor Frankl

This book has been quite a journey, hasn't it? But the journey is really just starting. What I asked from you at the beginning of this book was to just stick with me through it to the end. I didn't ask for you to trust me. I didn't ask for you to believe me. All I asked is that we be partners, that we walk through this together.

So you've reached the end now. What are you thinking? What do you want to do now? Do you want to go back to a treatment program that wasn't working? Perhaps if you just keep following along, doing what you've been doing, something will change. Maybe the next doctor will have the answers. Maybe the next protocol will be the secret formula. Or maybe not.

Wouldn't you rather launch yourself forward? Don't you want to reach a level you've never reached? What would it be like to take this leap of faith? To take your health into your own hands and experience a shift in the whole field of energy within and around you?

The difference between biohacking compared to the conventional medical system is that biohacking is designed to work with the innate life force within you. Biohacking strategies are designed to address root causes and harness the healing power of the body.

Biohacking is a constant work in progress. It is an assessment that goes on daily, weekly, and monthly. You're not waiting for somebody else to tell you whether there's improvement. You can see the improvement, whether through your body's feedback or through analyzing personal data. You know when your sleep is improving; you know when you feel less fatigue and more energy. Those things are measurable for yourself.

When you see or feel improvement, that's the momentum you need for recovery. That's what gets your body energized. That's what increases your vibration and creates a higher state of health. So as you track your progress, you get more and more excited about it. You actually see the results of your treatments, and you know its leading to the improvement you desire.

When you set your sights on improvement, all you want is to see more and more of that. Then you know you're on the right track. You know your actions are making a positive difference. Over the course of weeks and months, they're getting you to the next level of health. You see things working, and it gives you a boost. It's what keeps your momentum going.

Biohacking gives you the ability to stick with things that work and change course when it's clear something doesn't work. Have you wasted a whole bunch of time and energy following along with treatments or strategies that weren't working? I'm sure you have.

The idea behind biohacking is to constantly be assessing for yourself so that you can be on top of the situation. You don't rely on somebody else to make that assessment for you. When you give yourself that kind of decision-making power, you increase your sense of agency. You don't feel like you're at the whim of somebody else's opinion. You trust your body's feedback.

Biohacking is all about harnessing our greatest potential. It's about taking the intelligence already within our bodies and accelerating those processes to work on our behalf. It's about believing we are worthy of health, freedom, and the autonomy to choose for ourselves.

If you are ready to embrace this empowered way of being in the world, you are ready for biohacking. I believe in your individual greatness. I believe you are meant to thrive, not just survive. You were meant to become the badass this journey will help you become.

When you take leaps of faith, you become stronger and braver. You become more willing to take risks in all areas of your life. You start to see yourself in a whole new light. What other goals do you have? What else do you want from your relationships, lifestyle, work, and hobbies? When you start to take action in your health, it gives you an idea of what else is possible.

When we take action, we can transform the things in our lives we really want to change. Taking action affirms that something is deserving of our attention, time, and resources. It's how we show what we value, what something is really worth to us. When it comes to recovering from Lyme, you're either going to take radical action or you're not. That's your choice.

All I can tell you is that you were put on this planet to thrive. We really do need you here. Please give this your all. No one else can bring the gifts you've been given. You are a unique creation. So, please, for the sake of the rest of us, fight for your life. Stop at nothing to get well. We want you here. We need you here.

Now is the time to claim your health. Now is the time to put faith in yourself and dive into the life you deserve. The good news is that you can get well. When you truly believe that, you can heal. You don't need anything more than you already have inside you. I promise you.

You are more than ready to be a biohacker. You can do this! I'm here for you. Please reach out if you need support or encouragement. I am here, and I believe in you with all my heart.

AFTERWORD

"What we need is more people who specialize in the impossible."

—Theodore Roosevelt

I wrote this book because I know that so many people with Lyme are not getting well. What I desire most is to see these amazing, strong, capable individuals rise up beyond the challenges they are experiencing on a daily basis. What I want is to support these people I care so deeply about. I want to see them become victorious in their own right.

My world was small and dark for such a long time. I couldn't give love to anyone else the way I wanted to. I was caring for my body. I was caring for my psyche. I was just surviving. When you are in survival mode, all you can do is pay attention to your basic needs.

You can't give attention beyond that. You can't love others the way you really want to. You can't support them because you're giving your body all the attention it needs to heal. That's all you have inside you at that moment. And that's how it should be when you are healing.

But what I envision is a world in which people are helping each other. We desperately need a planet with far more healthy people. When people are healthy, they can take care of others. They can take care of the planet's resources. They can bring love, hope, and compassion to others.

Biohacking is a way people can become healthier. As we heal from illness and work to improve the condition of our bodies, we ultimately improve the condition of the whole planet. When we embrace this vision of possibility, we have a greater sense of purpose.

Illness is a continuum. It's an acceleration of our body's state of depletion. What's happening in our bodies shows us what is happening on a planetary level. Our bodies are inundated with too many toxins and chemicals that are stressing the immune system. We must make a change.

We need to make a commitment to creating a world that supports our human biology and our planet's ecology. Biohacking is a way to improve our bodies, our minds, and our spirits. It is a way to take back control of our own well-being and that of our greater society. This is our future.

I wrote this book because it's the book I needed; it's the one I'm still following every day. This is a new way of thinking. It's a different paradigm for life. It's a program for taking responsibility for your health, for your habits, and for all of your choices. When you follow this paradigm, you will have more joy, energy, and vitality. You will help to create a brave new world.

READER THANK-YOU

I truly appreciate your taking the time to read my book. As a way to express my gratitude, I'd love to give you a free list of biohacking strategies I used to treat Lyme disease and improve my health. Please contact me at www.beyondlyme.coach, and I will send it today!

Lastly, if you've found this book beneficial and encouraging, please share it somehow. Leaving a review on Amazon or Goodreads could help someone else launch to the next level of their healing journey. Together we can build up the biohacking community and spread the word!

ACKNOWLEDGMENTS

It's an absolute joy to honor the legions of people who have been a part of my journey. The hero's path is always lighted by supernatural aid, and I've witnessed that along my own path. Help has come at every step. Neither my recovery nor this book would've been possible without all the support I've received.

Thank you to my whole family, both in the seen and unseen worlds, for being my greatest fans. I'd like to recognize my grandmother Marlene Rainman, who was a scientist long before the time women were empowered to pursue their passions in research and medicine. Her fierce independence and scientific mind are a big part of who I am. Even though we weren't close during her time on earth, I feel intimately connected to her now. I thank her for paving the way for the women of the future to step into their power.

Enormous gratitude goes to my grandfather R. Paul Toeppen, for the benevolent patriarch he is. At one hundred years old, he is my greatest living inspiration and always will be. He made it possible for me to pursue innovative therapies, invest in biohacking tools, and prioritize my health despite lacking adequate insurance coverage for Lyme treatment in the broken medical system. He is a true survivor himself, having recovered from prostate cancer in his seventies, being in a coma due to a life-threatening infection in his eighties, and undergoing a colectomy at ninety. Doing Pilates daily and riding a stationary bike to stay strong at age one hundred, he motivates me to have his level of determination and dignity.

For championing me during the hardest times and supporting me as I enter a new phase in my life, I'd like to thank my immediate and extended family: my husband, Geoff, for standing alongside me with unconditional love and forgiveness while sacrificing so much of his life during the years of significant trauma; my mom, Stephanie, for strapping herself in beside me on the roller coaster of life and being a true mama bear; my nieces and nephews, Lauren, Kate, Griffin, Kyle and Ethan, for delighting me with your sweetness, humor, exuberance, creativity, Facetime calls, hugs, dance parties, and happy memories; my brother and sister-in-law, Scott and Jen, for loving me through the difficult years when I was really sick with Lyme and always having heartfelt concern for my health; my brother-in-law and sister-in-law, Jonathan and Danielle, for your empathy and teaching me that emotion can be expressed through the perfect music choices; my father, Mike, who supported my education and the writing of this book; my father-in-law, Gary, for always being so good-natured and asking about me; my uncle, Peter, and my "bonus dad," Roger, for being examples of thoughtful and expressive men; and for all of my aunts, uncles, and cousins from the Toeppen and Rudy clans (of which there are too many to name), for giving me dynamic energy.

I'd like to convey my deepest gratitude for the two people who truly pushed me to see myself beyond Lyme, living out my dreams for the future: my physician, Dr. Christine Schaffner, and my dear friend, Nicola Vitkovich. These two visionary women have been inspiring examples to me. They have created their own successful businesses, dealt with personal challenges along the way, and are totally devoted to their patients / clients. Thank you to my forever friends, Kristen and Amanda, for supporting me from a distance. These strong women are examples to me as well—being dedicated to science and justice. Gratitude to my friends and fellow health warriors, Katie, Daiva, Marie, Kamille, Melissa, Annie, and Chris, for sharing your journeys. Many thanks to the Gary Way neighborhood from my childhood for pulling for me. I'm so grateful to my friends, Greg and Shelley Krohn, for being the best neighbors I could ask for.

Thank you to my doctors and the staff at the Sophia Health Institute in Woodinville, Washington, for being so heartfelt in the practice of authentic health care: Dr. Dietrich Klinghardt, Dr. Christine Schaffner, Dr. Kara Nakisbendi, Destiny Chirls, Kim Yri, Kimmie Vetkos, Kim Todd, Eva Christenson, Jagna Larson, Nava Weigert,

Nidhi Niak, Cora Byers, Chloe Creasy, and Kelly Moore. A big thank-you to past Sophia staff and to Tiffany Sells for her devoted service to my needs as a patient. For taking such good care of me during many hours of intravenous infusions, I'd like to thank my nurses at the Envita Medical Center in Scottsdale, Arizona; the Desert Oasis Clinic in Las Vegas, Nevada; and the Holtorf Medical Group in El Segundo, California. I'd also like to thank Dr. Petra Dorfsman at Elysia Life Care in Santa Monica, California, for being an investigative doctor. Thanks to Daisy White for being a caring consultant.

Many thanks to all my healers for caring for my body through the most difficult circumstances: my lymphatic therapists, Laurie D'Andrea, Kristy Schaefl, Emi Calva-Terada, Maren Collins, Linda Birch, Ida Friedman, Susan Barrett, and Marchelle Brown; my bodyworkers and colon hydrotherapists at the Tummy Temple in Seattle, Heidi Ochsner, Janell Hartman, Tobyanna Everhart, Lauren Mulvery, and Mindy Meyer; my chiropractors, Dr. Steve Jacobsen, Dr. Cheree Sandness, Dr. Matthew Rivera, and the Joint Chiropractic; my Healing Touch practitioner, Vickie Smith; my brainspotting facilitator, Dr. Bruce Davis; my energy-work facilitator, Gregg Kirk; my family constellation facilitator, Andreanna Rainville; and my EMDR therapist, Don Elium.

Many thanks to all the individuals and professional organizations who are helping to educate the world about Lyme and support people in need. I'd especially like to thank Scott Forsgren for providing a true service through his many years as the Better Health Guy. He has shared a wealth of information with the Lyme community, and I honor him for all the work he's done. Many thanks to the physicians, scientists, researchers, and other healthcare professionals who are a part of the International Lyme and Associated Diseases Society (ILADS), the Academy of Comprehensive Integrative Medicine (ACIM), the Forum for Integrative Medicine (TFIM), the American Academy of Environmental Medicine (AAEM), and/or the American College for Advancement in Medicine (ACAM) for advancing our collective understanding of Lyme and other complex diseases. I also want to highlight the Lymelight Foundation for their generosity in providing patients with grants for treatment support.

Many thanks to scientific and medical pioneers for the information they've put out into the world: Dr. Daniel Amen, Dr. Shawn Baker, Dr. William Bengston, Dr. Ed Breitschwerdt, Stephen Buhner, Dr. Natasha Campbell-McBride, Dr. Lee Cowden, Dr. Jennifer Daniels, Dr. James DiNicolantonio, Dr. Joe Dispenza, Dr. Norman Doidge, Dr. Hartmut Fischer, Dr. Jason Fung, Jim Humble, Dr. Andreas Kalcker, Dr. Doug Kaufmann, Dr. Bessel Van der Kolk, Dr. Walter Last, Dr. Bruce Lipton, Dr. Joseph Mercola, Dr. Judy Mikovits, Dr. Robert Mozayeni, Dr. Antje Oswald, Dr. William Pawluk, Dr. Daniel Pompa, Dr. Kerri Rivera, Dr. Paul Saladino, Dr. Stephanie Seneff, Dr. Thomas Seyfried, Dr. Christopher Shade, Dr. Angela Stanton, Dr. Jerry Tennant, Dr. John Trowbridge, Dr. Louisa Williams, Dr. Alex Volinsky, and Dr. Simon Yu.

For inspiring me to embrace the field of biohacking in my own way, I'd like to thank Dave Asprey and his podcast Bulletproof Radio, which supplied me with many hundreds of hours of learning during the years of detox and self-care. As founder of Upgrade Labs and the annual Biohacking Conference in Southern California, Dave has set an example of what is possible when like-minded biohackers share within a community.

I'd like to thank my Human Potential Institute tribe for all of the training, coaching collaboration, and personal development I've received. A huge thanks to my instructors and mentors Ronit Lemon, Rod Francis, Val Jennings, and Dr. Mark Atkinson, for teaching me to be a good coach. Many thanks to my fellow Human Potential colleagues for continuing to support one another and grow the field of coaching.

This book has been quite an interesting process of evolution. Thank you to Dr. Christine Schaffner and Dr. Kara Nakisbendi for encouraging me to write it. I'm grateful to my coaches, Katie Hollenkamp, Karin Reed, and Dr. Kathryn Guylay for helping me to focus on my efforts toward this goal and pursue action steps to achieve it. For their editing support, I'd like to thank Andrae Smith, Nkechi Obi, and Moriah Richard. A tremendous thanks goes to my managing editor, Michele Preisendorf, at Eschler Editing. I deeply appreciate everything you have done to make this project a success. I'd also like to thank my audiobook producer, Daryl Bolicek, at Wild Horse Recording, for making the listening experience into something amazing. I am so grateful for all of you!

ABOUT THE AUTHOR

Lisa Rudy Williams is a personal coach, biohacking consultant, and alternative health educator. Her mission is to empower individuals to take bold action on their goals and experiment with open-minded curiosity in every area of their life. With her background in science, research, and neurobiology, she brings a unique perspective to helping her clients.

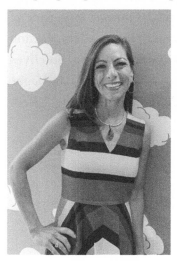

Having battled back from the brink of late-stage Lyme disease, co-infections, and other major health challenges, Lisa is poised to help those who are ready to confidently move ahead with their own journey to better health. Through her programs, she provides one-on-one and group coaching along with consulting to motivated clients. She has earned coaching certifications from the Life Purpose Institute and Human Potential Institute. She's also accredited by the International Coaching Federation as an Associate Certified Coach.

Lisa earned her bachelor's degree in cognitive science with a concentration in neuroscience from the University of Virginia. She spent several years as a clinical research associate with the Amen Clinics Inc., studying brain function and conducting research studies. She later became a high school biology teacher and then a personal trainer. Her education and understanding of the inseparable unity of the brain and body are an important part of her work.

Lisa's love of sunflowers, convertibles cars, Broadway musicals, kids craft projects, sports, the mountains, Karen Drucker songs, and bright colors might make her seem like an unlikely biohacker. Lisa is committed to her health because she wants to pursue a lifetime of hobbies, like hiking, swimming, cycling, dancing, skiing, kayaking, paddleboarding, and scuba diving. She lives amid red rocks and wide-open spaces in Las Vegas, Nevada, with her husband, Geoff, and their dog, Leia.

Made in the USA
Monee, IL
19 August 2020